D0901109

CBD

FOR THE VESTIBULAR
PATIENT

CBD

For The Vestibular Patient

Mark Knoblauch PhD

Kiremma Press
Houston, TX

© 2020 by Mark Knoblauch

All rights reserved. No part of this book may be reproduced or used in any manner without the express written permission of the author or publisher except for the use of brief quotations in a book review.

Printed in the United States of America

Disclaimer: The information provided within this book is for general informational purposes only. While the author has tried to keep the information up-to-date and correct, there are no representations or warranties, express or implied, about the completeness, accuracy, reliability, suitability or availability with respect to the information contained in this book for any purpose. Any use of this information is at your own risk. At no time is any material within this book intended to represent or substitute for sound medical advice. Furthermore, the methods described within this book are the author's personal thoughts and opinions. As such, they are not intended to be a definitive set of instructions or recommendations for you to follow precisely. You may discover there are other methods and materials to accomplish the same end result.

To all those who have to live with the misery of a vestibular disorder and to those who are working to find ways to lessen every vestibular disorder's impact

Table of Contents

Foreword xi

Introduction xi

Chapter 1 – The basics of cannabis 15

    A brief background 15

    Cannabis-associated terminology 17

        A plant by any other name 17

        Cannabis derivative terminology 20

    Cannabis market 22

    Anatomy of the cannabis plant 22

    Legal aspects of cannabis 25

        Evolving trends 27

    Why regulate? 31

    Conclusion 32

Chapter 2 – The Vestibular System 37

    Sections of the ear 38

        Outer ear 38

        Middle ear 38

        Inner ear..39

    The vestibular system 41

            Saccule...44

            Utricle..45

        Semicircular Canals...46

    Vertigo and the vestibular system 49

    The vestibulo-ocular reflex (VOR) 51

Conclusion 53

Chapter 3 – The Endocannabinoid System 57

Background of the endocannabinoid system 58

Endocannabinoids 60

Phytocannabinoids 61

Cannabinoid receptors 62

    The CB1 receptor 62

    The CB2 receptor 65

Terpenes 66

A perplexing system 68

Medical effects of cannabinoids 69

Conclusion 71

Chapter 4 – Cannabidiol 75

The basics of CBD 75

Market presence of CBD 77

Defining the cannabidiol user 77

Safety and side effects of CBD 78

    Side effects of CBD 80

Potential Drug Interactions 82

CBD and THC 84

Effects of CBD 85

Misconceptions of CBD Effects 88

Labeling Accuracy 90

The CBD extraction process 95

    CO_2 extraction 98

    Solvent Extraction 98

    Ice Water Extraction 99

Oil Extraction 99

CBD Delivery methods 100

    Topical application 101

    Drops or sprays 102

    Edibles (including pills) 102

    Inhalation 102

CBD dosing 103

Conclusion 108

Chapter 5 – Finding a quality CBD source .. 115

What to look for in your CBD 116

Conclusion 121

Chapter 6 – The Scientific Process 123

Why we need the scientific process 124

    Testing on subjects 127

    True effects vs coincidence 130

    Designing experiments 131

    Summarizing the scientific process 135

Conclusion 136

Chapter 7 – CBD and Vestibular Conditions 139

Tinnitus 140

    CBD and Tinnitus 142

Ménière's disease 143

    CBD and Ménière's 144

Benign paroxysmal positional vertigo 144

    CBD and BPPV 145

Vestibular migraine 146

    CBD and Vestibular Migraine 147

Persistent Postural-Perceptual Dizziness (PPPD).... 148

    CBD and PPPD.. 149

Vestibular neuritis.. 149

    CBD and vestibular neuritis................................. 150

Acoustic Neuroma.. 150

    Acoustic Neuroma and CBD 151

    Conclusion 151

Conclusion **157**

Glossary 163

Appendix A. Drug Schedules................................. 169

Foreword

When Mark Knoblauch first asked if I would consider writing the foreword for his most recent book, *CBD For The Vestibular Patient*, I thought "why not"? I can easily put a few paragraphs together and say some nice things about the book. After all, Dr. Knoblauch is a professional colleague of mine whom I have come to highly respect over the past few years of interacting with him.

After having read the book, all I can say is "wow"! If I were patient suffering from a vestibular disorder and trying to find anything to make me feel better – I have just found a gem. Dr. Knoblauch is a captivating writer who has a talent for simplifying the complicated. In this, his 15th book, he doesn't disappoint. In just the last few years alone the hype over CBD as some form of magic cure for every ailment has consumed nearly every industry in one way or another. How does one know the truth about what CBD can and cannot do? Why not give it a try if you haven't found a satisfactory solution to your vestibular disorder? Well, simply grasping for the straw that contains the CBD tipping point is not likely a well thought out plan for success. In fact, it is more likely a willing stretch at the expense of hard-earned dollars. This doesn't mean that CBD does not work or that it can't be of help for vestibular disorders.

The service that Dr. Knoblauch has done for every person wondering if CBD can help resolve or keep under control one's vestibular disorder cannot be underestimated. When only 62% of pharmacy schools and 9% of medical schools report in 2019 teaching students about cannabis in their curriculums the patient is left to become more of an educated consumer than ever before. This is not an easy place to be. It makes sense that before any medicinally promoted product become available to the general public for health benefits that is stands the test of scrutiny as it relates to potential benefits and risks, side effects, addictive properties, etc. We call this evidence. We live in an evidence-based world where we must justify what we do based upon sound scientific research. Why is CBD different? Why is there consumer pressure on state and federal governments to legalize all forms of cannabis before it is ever properly tested? Are we not worried and concerned about risks of putting something on or in our bodies without knowing the potential harm it could have? Or are we less concerned with that and driven more by finding the quickest solution to our problem that has not been solved over decades and centuries of existing and extensive research?

It took me just a few hours to read through the book from cover to cover. I tried to do so by putting myself in your shoes – the patient with a vestibular disorder wanting to know if CBD will be of any help. As noted, there isn't a simple answer, nor is there a single answer. Understanding the cannabis genus plant and all that it contains paints a much clearer picture of what CBD actually is beyond a catchy acronym. Knowing how it is proposed to interact with the body based upon dosage, application, and receptor binding is helpful to know. If you are reading this, you likely already have a good understanding of the vestibular system. The ability to connect the dots between the vestibular system and the endocannabinoid system allow you to become an educated patient. Perhaps most importantly, the advice given in the book about finding quality CBD products and evaluating the evidence behind each is a skill set that each and every patient should possess regardless of what one's personal medical condition is.

In *CBD For The Vestibular Patient* Dr. Knoblauch captures all of the critical pieces of information required for the patient with a vestibular disorder to make an educated decision about his or her use of CBD as a treatment intervention. The content is timely, informative, and easily understood for any person to benefit from. Dr. Knoblauch lays out the history of CBD, the current research and lack thereof, and the opportunities that lie ahead for future findings. In short, *CBD For The Vestibular Patient* is a must read!

Jeff G. Konin, PhD, ATC, PT, FACSM, FNATA
Clinical Professor, Florida International University
President & Founder, PHD420, Inc.
www.PhD420.org

Introduction

Until you've had one of the many vestibular-related conditions, it's hard to understand the degree of impact that a small disruption to one's vestibular system can have. Dizziness, tinnitus, vertigo, nausea, and nystagmus are symptoms that most everyone has experienced at some point, but for vestibular patients these symptoms can often be unending. Hours of lying in bed trapped by a vertigo attack or being unable to walk down a grocery store aisle due to sudden imbalance often become a part of life. When you couple these symptoms with factors such as anxiety, social withdrawal, and repeated last-minute cancellations, the true extent of life with a vestibular disorder can be understood.

For many individuals, one of the worst aspects of living with a vestibular condition comes in the form of people often telling you that you 'look fine'. Sure, we look fine, but the very definition of a symptom is that it is an event which must be reported by the patient as it cannot be seen by an outsider. Therefore, we're left dealing with the inner torment of vestibular hell while exhibiting few outward signs. And when one's life becomes so overwhelmed with the effects of a vestibular disorder, patients are often willing to try whatever means necessary to achieve relief. Whereas prescriptions or traditional treatments rarely provide relief, patients are left to decide whether less proven techniques, treatments, or medicines are worth trying.

The growth of social media over the past 20 years could be considered quite a boon to patients as it provides a source of information as well as a way to interact with those who have similar medical issues. Private groups, forums, and dedicated websites can provide a wealth of information and are often tailored specifically for individual disorders such as vestibular migraine or acoustic neuroma. However, social media might also be considered to have opened up a unique set of problems for patients as its 'open-access' nature can often allow anyone to get involved regardless of expertise, credentials, or evidence of accuracy. This in turn can often lead to patients being exposed to quite a bit of anecdotal information rather than science-based evidence. For the vestibular patient looking for any available option to stop the misery of their symptoms, it can be extremely difficult to separate fact from anecdote amidst the expanse that social media has become.

The attention afforded to cannabis-based products has grown extensively over the past decade in the United States. As more interest becomes focused toward cannabis from the science and medical fields, coupled with its growing legalization, medical patients have taken note of the potential benefits that cannabis and its derivatives may be able to provide for them. Cannabidiol (CBD), a cannabis derivative, has itself exhibited a surge of interest from the medical field in the past few years. While claims on social media indicate that CBD can seemingly fix everything from skin rashes to severe vertigo, it can be tough for patients to be able to sift through the wealth of claims in order to establish fact from fiction. When coupled with the fact that CBD – like all cannabis-based products – is still highly regulated by the government and therefore remains limited in its ability to be studied, patients can feel as though they are left in a figurative vacuum between the fascinating claims about cannabis products' potential benefits and the fact that it lacks extensive evidence from the scientific community. To some, this lack of scientific evidence for CBD as a potential treatment option can invite issues such as skepticism, misunderstanding, and false hope from some hardened individuals who demand solid evidence for its effectiveness. Unfortunately, establishing the true effects of any product through the process of empirical research can take years – years that many vestibular patients are not willing to wait.

Therein lies the purpose of this book – to both sort through the relevant scientific research on CBD in order to provide a fact-based set of information for you or those you know who have vestibular disorders, and also to identify the basis for CBD as a potential treatment option for vestibular disorders. In effect, you can view this book as serving to provide a foundation of what CBD is and how it works which will then allow you to decide if it's best for you and your medical condition. What you will not find in this book is any upselling or bias. I am not looking to sell you a product because I don't promote any product. Nor will I ask you to pay a monthly membership fee to my website for more information. Like all my vestibular books, my intent as an author is only to provide you factual information that you can then use to make the best health-based decisions for yourself.

To do this, we'll first take a look in Chapter 1 at the basics of cannabis, where we'll briefly outline its history, discuss some of the more common cannabis-related terminology used, and then look at the regulation associated with cannabis, marijuana, and hemp use. Next, we'll switch gears to outline the basic anatomy and physiology of the vestibular system with the intent of providing you a primer into how the vestibular system works. Then in Chapter 3 we'll transition over to detailing the basics of the endocannabinoid system that CBD specifically interacts with. We'll then use that information to set up Chapter 4's focus on cannabidiol itself where we'll look at a variety of topics including safety and side effects, known effects of CBD, and extraction methods used to obtain CBD. We'll look in Chapter 5 at a few recommendations for you to consider when you look to purchase CBD. Chapter 6 will focus on helping you to be able to evaluate the available evidence so that you can decipher the vast amount of information and recommendations you may hear from friends and family as well as on social media. Finally, Chapter 7 will address some of the more common vestibular conditions while also identifying any known CBD-related research for each of the discussed conditions.

My goal is that upon having read this book you have a greater understanding of the vestibular system, what cannabis and its main derivatives are, how the endocannabinoid system works, and what research has revealed specific to the effects of cannabis and its derivatives on the vestibular system. Certainly, we don't cover 'everything' in this book; rather, I tried to draw out the most pertinent information to provide you a solid foundation toward understanding the basics of CBD as a vestibular patient. There are literally chapters of information that could be added, and finding a stopping point for each chapter proved difficult. Quite frankly, this book could have easily been written as a brief introductory guide for CBD users, but I felt that relating it more toward vestibular conditions would help you better understand the relationship between CBD and potential treatments for your own vestibular conditions.

With that being said, let's get started down the path of learning whether CBD may be a beneficial treatment option for you.

Chapter 1 – The basics of cannabis

E ven though you're reading a book that focuses on cannabidiol as a therapy, it's worthwhile for us to first step back and outline cannabis, the main source of cannabidiol. Much like it probably isn't productive to have a discussion about vestibular migraine without first outlining the vestibular system as well as how balance is processed in the brain, I don't personally believe that you can truly understand cannabidiol until you've learned a bit about cannabis. Therefore, this chapter is designed to orient you to the properties of the cannabis plant itself, with special attention focused on those aspects that directly relate to cannabidiol.

A brief background

People have been harnessing the purported medical benefits of cannabis for over 5,000 years. Originally thought to have been localized to central Asia, eventually, with the assistance of human intervention, cannabis evolved to thrive throughout much of the globe[1]. During this early time, cannabis was used predominantly as a food source, as a source of material fiber, and as a source of medicine, while becoming recognized for its drug capacity only in the last century[2].

As a medicine, cannabis has quite a storied history. Inhabitants of ancient China used extracts of cannabis to treat pain and muscle cramps[3] yet also took advantage of cannabis's ability to "take away the mind" when used in excess[4]. Later, stone carvings from around 2350 B.C. revealed the first documented use of cannabis for medicinal purposes[4]. Many years later, cannabis gained used as a treatment for nocturnal epilepsy, providing us an early hint into what was later discovered to be the anticonvulsant properties of cannabis[4].

As the 1800s rolled around, the muscle-relaxant capabilities of cannabis were recognized, thereby providing a viable treatment option for tetanus[5]. Cannabis eventually made it into the United States Pharmacopeia in 1850 based on its use with conditions such as cholera, rabies, gout, insanity, and tetanus, among others[6]. Cannabis even found its way into the ingredient list of many medicines during this time, providing a strong indication of its alleged medicinal qualities[2].

Because of the purported beneficial effects of cannabis, interest was developed toward establishing its therapeutic makeup. This interest eventually led to the discovery of one of its components, Δ9-trans-(6aR,10aR)-tetrahydrocannabinol, or "THC". Later, based largely on what is considered by many to be propaganda and other scare tactics associated with the psychogenic aspect of cannabis use, the Marijuana Tax Act of 1937 was enacted to criminalize cannabis use and effectively ban cannabis sales. Eventually, the Marihuana Tax Act was replaced in the 1970s by the Controlled Substances Act[7] that remains in place to this day.

Fast-forward to the present, and nearly 500 compounds and over 100 cannabinoids have been identified from cannabis[8]. Advancements in technology as well as our understanding of biochemistry are slowly but surely revealing key mechanisms into the makeup of cannabis specific to how it affects our body. Hopefully, as improvements in technology and biochemistry continue, we will be able to gain further insight into the potential benefits of cannabis, particularly how it can improve several of the vestibular disorders that exist.

Cannabis-associated terminology

Visit enough websites or read enough research and you'll quickly learn that there is a wealth of unique terminology thrown around specific to cannabis and its associated derivatives. Unfortunately, a lack of consistency in the cannabis world probably contributes to some of the confusion that is often connected with cannabis-related terms. Next, we'll look at some of the more common terminology that we'll be using in this book as well as what you'll come across when navigating the cannabidiol world. Also, be sure to check out the glossary near the end of this book as it expands into much more of the associated terminology.

Let's start with the basics. Probably the most foundational term to grasp is *cannabis,* a word which comes from *cannabacaea* that represents a family of about 170 individual flowering plants. Cannabis is the genus of hemp plant that includes several varieties such as *cannabis sativa, cannabis indica, and cannabis ruderalis.* The well-known term *marijuana* (or *marihuana* in some older literature) is intimately related to these varieties as it is the more commonly used name for the *cannabis sativa* variety[9]. As we'll learn later, however, 'marijuana' as a plant description is actually associated more with THC content than a specific variety of plant.

A plant by any other name . . .

We have to pause here a minute and put a bit of focus into the terms *cannabis, hemp,* and *marijuana.* At first glance amongst

17

the literature, they are relatively representative of the same thing – the cannabis plant. The term 'marijuana' probably has a more sinister association with illicit use, while 'cannabis' may conjure up the same ideas among some people yet is generally more associated with scientific-use aspects of the *cannabis sativa* plant. The term 'hemp' is typically connected more with aspects such as textile production, though its close association with marijuana and cannabis may be a source of confusion.

It might be somewhat surprising to learn that according to some, the end purpose of the plant can determine which name it gets assigned. With this approach, however, the vast array of uses for the plant serves to introduce additional terminology. The cannabis plant is often designated as "hemp" when it is being used for its fiber but called "hempseed" when harvesting the plant for seed oil[10]. Designating the plant as hemp may induce further classifications, as "industrial hemp" refers to specific domesticated strains of the plant that are grown specifically for fiber or oil and are not cultivated for psychedelic products. "Marijuana" is a term typically applied to the cannabis plant when the end result of production is for a drug-related (recreational and/or pharmaceutical) or psychogenic purpose.

While that may help clarify the proper terminology, the U.S. government provides a bit more specific definition regarding the terms 'hemp' versus 'marijuana', clarifying that specific *parts* of the plant largely determine the proper terminology. Hemp, for example, is described according to Section 297A of the Agricultural Marketing Act of 1946 as[11]:

" . . . the plant Cannabis sativa L. and any part of that plant, including the seeds thereof and all derivatives, extracts, cannabinoids, isomers, acids, salts, and salts of isomers, whether growing or not, with a delta-9 tetrahydrocannabinol [delta-9 THC] concentration of not more than 0.3 percent on a dry weight basis."

Marijuana, on the other hand, is defined by (21 U.S.C. §802(16)) as:

> ". . . all parts of the plant Cannabis sativa L, whether growing or not; the seeds thereof; the resin extracted from any part of such plant; and every compound, manufacture, salt, derivative, mixture, or preparation of such plant, its seeds or resin. Such term does not include the mature stalks of such plant, fiber produced from such stalks, oil or cake made from the seeds of such plant, any other compound, manufacture, salt, derivative, mixture, or preparation of such mature stalks (except the resin extracted therefrom), fiber, oil, or cake, or the sterilized seed of such plant which is incapable of germination"

Therefore, according to the U.S. government, the classification of hemp from marijuana is dependent upon the *part* of the plant utilized as well as ensuring that hemp does not contain more than 0.3% THC. The government does not, however, differentiate the term cannabis from marijuana or hemp other than to state that hemp and marijuana are distinct 'forms' of cannabis which includes all of its industrial, medicinal, and recreational varieties[11].

The variety of cannabis-related names and classifications can certainly be confusing, and media or online literature interchange of these terms are quite common. Not surprisingly, the industrial hemp industry is putting forth a strong effort to make it clear to the public that "hemp is not marijuana."[10]. As regulations likely ease more in the future, it is hoped that proper terminology gains traction so as to better differentiate the specific use of the cannabis plant and its products.

Cannabis derivative terminology

Because future chapters will be largely looking at the effects that cannabis derivatives such as CBD can have on our body, we have to take a moment to outline these derivatives as well. Existing within our individual cell membranes are specific proteins called *receptors* that bind to a unique set of messenger molecules known as *cannabinoids*. Cannabinoids that are present within our body are known as *endocannabinoids* – short for 'endogenous cannabinoids' – and represent that group of cannabinoids that are produced within our body. Endocannabinoids are one component of our *endocannabinoid system* that is also comprised of *endogenous* (i.e. 'from within the body') *cannabinoids* as well as the associated receptors and enzymes. *Exogenous* (i.e. 'from outside of the body') *cannabinoids* are also detected by our endocannabinoid system yet are comprised of any cannabinoid introduced to the body from an external source – such as through the use of cannabis or one of its derivatives.

While endocannabinoids are produced by and used within our body to activate cannabinoid receptors, *phytocannabinoids* (*phyto* = plant) are produced within plants. Despite being produced outside of our body, the structure and chemical makeup of a phytocannabinoid allows it to bind to specific receptors within our body's endocannabinoid system and generate the same effects as an endocannabinoid. Originally, the term phytocannabinoid represented only cannabis-related cannabinoids. Now, however, the term has been revised to represent any plant-based molecule capable of interacting with cannabinoid receptors[12].

To be clear, regardless of the cannabinoid source (i.e. endo- vs. phyto-), when a cannabinoid binds to an endocannabinoid system receptor it triggers that receptor to start an action that causes a physiological event such as

20

phosphorylation or release of a particular neurotransmitter. It does not matter whether the triggering cannabinoid was of endo- or phytocannabinoid origin as both are capable of binding to and activating the cannabinoid receptor.

The literature seems to invite some confusion that the name 'cannabinoid' indicates that the molecule originates from cannabis plants, which is not necessarily true. The association between cannabis and receptors in our body actually occurred as a result of researchers trying to outline why THC caused its psychogenic effects. In the late 1980s, receptors were identified that would bind to THC and generate the subsequent effects[13]. This in turn led to a focused investigation into that receptor which over time led to our discovery of receptors that responded to cannabis – hence the 'cannabinoid' name – and revealed at last the endocannabinoid system. Thereafter, molecules that bind to receptors of the endocannabinoid system were classified as cannabinoids. It is important to understand that because they are capable of binding to our endocannabinoid system's receptor, phytocannabinoids have the same ability to cause a physiological action in our body as those endocannabinoids that our body produces. That ability explains why anandamide and cannabidiol are both classified as cannabinoids even though anandamide is produced within the body while cannabidiol is a product of the cannabis plant.

You have most likely heard much about the major psychoactive phytocannabinoid, THC. Perhaps surprisingly, THC is considered to be the most popular illegal chemical in the world, and it ranks fourth – behind caffeine, ethyl alcohol, and nicotine – among what are considered 'addictive' recreational chemicals[10]. Despite what is usually a bad rap for THC, it has been shown to have very beneficial qualities including acting as a bronchodilator and antioxidant as well as having over 20 times more anti-inflammatory effect than aspirin and two times more than hydrocortisone[14]! Unlike THC, however, phytocannabinoids such as cannabidiol and cannabigerol (CBG) do not have psychotropic (i.e. 'mind-altering') effects because of their inability to bind to the specific cannabinoid receptor responsible for generating the psychotropic effects[15].

Cannabis market

The market surrounding the cannabis plant is quite immense, and with a recent lessening of federal regulations regarding its use, the market should be expected to expand even more. In the United States, hemp-containing products reached $820 million in sales in 2017, with projections of nearly $2 billion by 2022[16]. Cannabidiol itself experienced a 57% market growth over the previous year, combining with hemp oil to reach $238 million in sales[17]. Even marijuana maintains a significant portion of the market, as marijuana is used by approximately 180 million people around the globe[18] and legal-use market sales are projected to reach $22 billion in 2020[19]. Despite its economic potential, the ongoing illicit drug market has largely stigmatized cannabis as the world's most recognizable, notorious and controversial plant[10].

Anatomy of the cannabis plant

Cannabis is considered to be an annual plant with an expected life cycle of up to seven months. Plants reach varying heights of 1-5 meters, with height ultimately dependent upon the particular cannabis variety (e.g. *cannabis sativa* vs. *cannabis indica*)[10]. While cannabinoids can be found in both male and female varieties, female cannabis plants have become the choice of cultivators due to their increased phytocannabinoid production as compared to male plants which tend to produce a much lower phytocannabinoid quantity[2].

Several inter-variety differences can be found between the more common *cannabis sativa* and *cannabis indica* varieties of plants. For example, a broader leaf structure is common to *cannabis indica* while a taller average height is reached in the *cannabis sativa* variety. Phytocannabinoid content has also been shown to differ between varieties, as *cannabis sativa* has little to no CBD while *cannabis indica* has been found to have considerable levels[10]. Even though the two plant types have been shown to have a unique genetic makeup, selective plant breeding has diminished those differences somewhat[20].

The structural makeup of the cannabinoid-producing portion of cannabis is somewhat consistent across varieties. Flowers from the cannabis plant are clustered into what are known as *buds,* and buds are typically found bunched together to form a physical structure known as a *cola* (Figure 1.1).

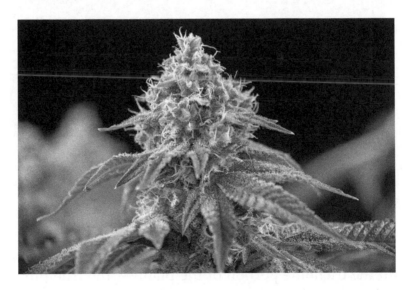

Figure 1.1. The main cola of the cannabis plant, shown here, typically grows at the top of the plant

Typically, a primary cola will form near the top of the stalk in budding plants, and phytocannabinoids as well as additional chemical components such as terpenes can be found in the unfertilized female flowers that make up the buds of the cannabis plant[21]. There, phytocannabinoids are produced within small bulbous projections found throughout the buds on what are known as glandular trichomes ('trichomes' would be considered as 'hairs' in mammals) (Figure 1.2).

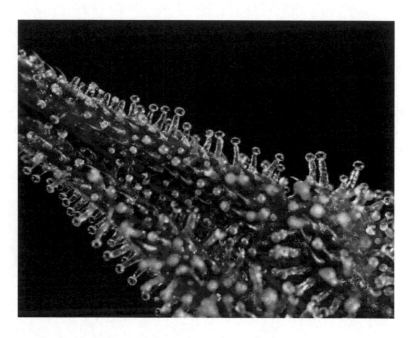

Figure 1.2. Present on each bud of the cannabis plant are thousands of small projections called trichomes that produce a resin containing several important chemicals of the cannabis plant such as cannabinoids and terpenes

Although phytocannabinoids are largely produced within the trichome portion of the plant[22], the true purpose of *why* phytocannabinoids are produced by the plant remains unclear[10]. It is theorized that cannabinoids evolved so as to provide protection against predators[2]. Evidence for this theory lies in the fact that certain phytocannabinoids can cause apoptosis (i.e. cell death) of insect cells[23]. Interestingly, insects themselves lack cannabinoid receptors[10], so a biological response to phytocannabinoids in insects similar to that which occurs with the endocannabinoid system in animals is not possible.

Different parts of the cannabis plant have varying amounts of phytocannabinoids, with the stems and older leaves having significantly lower levels than newer leaves and the female flowers. Age of the plant also factors into the phytocannabinoid content, as the amount within the cannabis plant has been shown to increase as the plant ages, ultimately reaching its highest amount at the plant's budding stage[2]. Along these same lines, the phytocannabinoid content of a plant can vary slightly in response to temperature, light intensity, and nutrients[10]. Ultimate retrievable cannabinoid content, however, is dependent upon cannabinoid extraction from the plant followed by chemical analysis of the extract. A discussion of the harvest and processing of cannabinoids from the cannabis plant will be discussed in a later chapter.

Legal aspects of cannabis

There's no question that anyone reading this book is at least familiar with the legal stigma that is ever-present with cannabis and cannabis use. If I were ever asked if there was a simple way to sum up the legalities associated with cannabis and cannabinoids, I would propose this one: *it's confusing.* The fact that marijuana is viewed as a controlled substance – and therefore illegal to possess – by the government is countered by recent changes to regulations involving hemp production. Although the regulations surrounding cannabis have lessened to the point that there is a slim sliver of legality that can be attained, the issue becomes further clouded in trying to stay within federal regulations and individual state laws. The confusion is complicated more by evidence that federal laws are usually not enforced in states that have legalized marijuana use[24], and that state regulations can differ widely based on whether the use is for medical or recreational use. Furthermore, medical-use allowances for marijuana differ based upon the state in which it is allowed. As a patient seeking medical benefits from cannabis, it can be dizzying to try and keep up with the laws as well as the ongoing changes to those laws. While an improvement in your condition is obviously the goal for using cannabis or its derivatives, doing so within the letter of the law can be challenging and may even make you wonder whether it's all worth it.

As a drug, the marijuana plant and its derivatives (e.g. cannabidiol) are federally regulated as controlled substances by the Controlled Substances Act. Consequently, there are a wealth of laws that anyone considering cannabis as a therapeutic drug or treatment must thoroughly evaluate. Because laws can change at any time across individual states in addition to what falls under federal regulations, it is important that you as a patient are aware of which regulations you are bound by, particularly what is most current – not just what might be found on a two-year-old website – because any relevant law, regulation, or even employment policy may have changed since the online information you found was originally posted.

In the next section we will talk briefly about some of the legal aspects of cannabis use specific to what you as a patient should be aware of regarding the associated regulations. This is *not* – and I strongly emphasize *__not__* – a guide to the legalities of cannabis or cannabinoid use either recreationally or medically, as several aspects discussed below are current only as of when they were printed in the literature and therefore may well have changed by the time you read this book. An understanding of the legalities of marijuana and its derivatives is a responsibility that lies with you the patient through collaboration with your medical provider, and it is imperative that you and your provider remain current as to the updated regulations specific to your own state and/or employment setting.

Evolving trends

Attitudes about the criminal aspect of marijuana have been waning. One survey revealed that the proportion of people who feel marijuana should *not* be legalized has dropped by 50% from 2000 – 2018[25]. One could guess that as regulations change, as stigmas are investigated, and as more research into the medical benefits of cannabis is performed, these beliefs will continue to decrease. Regardless, there's little dispute that cannabis use has been the source of intense debate for years. A battle has (and likely will continue to be) waged between the legal, legislative, and medical communities over the rationale behind maintaining strict cannabis regulations in light of potential medical benefits. As mentioned earlier, because of the ever-changing aspect of cannabis regulation, you as a patient must familiarize yourself with cannabis-related laws specific to your state and/or jurisdiction as well as the policies specific to your place of employment. To be clear, even employers are able to outline their own cannabis policies for the workplace as they operate under *federal* hiring guidelines; therefore, despite legal allowances by a state to use marijuana recreationally, an employee may still be fired in that state if the use is prohibited by a workplace policy[26].

In looking at regulations specific to medical marijuana use, acceptance of medical marijuana as a viable treatment appears to be gaining steam. For example, several states such as New York, Arizona, and Connecticut have enacted laws that prohibit an employer from discriminating against an employee who is using marijuana for medical purposes[27]. After all, it is often an intent with medical marijuana to achieve the therapeutic benefits (e.g. anti-nausea, pain relief) without specifically seeking the psychoactive effects. This very situation is what often drives the pursuit of cannabinoid research – to reveal additional medical benefits from cannabis without involving the mind-altering consequences brought about by THC. It will be of interest to observe whether still more states pursue a patient's legal right to use medical marijuana as further advancements in our understanding of its medical benefits become known.

Despite known medical benefits, cannabis remains a Schedule-1 drug according to the Controlled Substance Act of 1970 (see 'Appendix A' for an outline of the different drug schedules). This designation indicates that the government, according to the requirements of a Schedule-1 drug, views cannabis to have no medical benefit and a high potential for abuse. However, the controversy surrounding cannabis goes back much further. Since Harry Anslinger's 1937 Marihuana Tax Act, federal law has prohibited the use and distribution of marijuana in the United States. Not much changed politically until the mid-1990s, when personal beliefs finally began to influence marijuana's legal standing. California began the legislative movement when in 1996 it passed the Compassionate Use Act to allow for the use of medical marijuana in that state[28]. This initial push began an eventual movement by over 30 states, the District of Columbia, Puerto Rico, Guam, and the U.S. Virgin Islands in lessening laws to allow for medical marijuana use[29].

The move towards medical marijuana legalization likely played a role in relaxed laws towards recreational marijuana use as well. In 2012, Colorado and Washington became the first states to allow for recreational marijuana use, later followed by nine other states[29]. This ongoing trend toward changes in attitude regarding marijuana regulation is highlighted by data showing that since 2016, 26 states now allow for medical marijuana use while 21 states have decriminalized at least some marijuana offenses[30].

One major advancement regarding cannabis regulation and that of its derivatives came in 2014 with the passage of the Agriculture Act[31], known unofficially as the 2014 "Farm Bill". This Act had a major effect on the cannabis industry, specifically regarding the hemp plant[32]. Through legislation written into the Farm Bill, hemp effectively became a crop. In addition, the regulations around the use of CBD were lessened, though not specifically legalized. For example, hemp-derived cannabinoids are made legal under the Farm Bill if certain conditions are met. Specifically, as long as the hemp is grown and processed under the stipulations of the Farm Bill as well as under individual state and federal regulations, and the hemp is cultivated by a licensed hemp grower, the produced CBD is considered legal. However, failure to meet one or more of the Farm Bill's requirements specific to hemp cultivation ensures that the cultivated cannabinoid will remain illegal as set out by federal law.

Medical marijuana plays into the changing ideals behind cannabis use, as many states have enacted laws specific to marijuana that is used for medicinal purposes, and within certain conditions[33]. Of particular interest in this area was that in 2009, the United States Attorney General announced that federal authorities would stop interfering with medical marijuana dispensaries, so long as those locations were operating in compliance with state laws[24]. This hands-off approach from the federal government led to a rapid increase in medical marijuana registration among patients in states with related laws[28]. Still, states such as Nebraska, Idaho, and South Dakota do not currently have any *cannabis sativa* access laws, which thereby makes CBD sale or consumption illegal in those states[31].

Despite the Farm Bill's relaxing of regulations, the legality of CBD in the United States is still confusing to many. Whereas CBD is classified as a 'new' medicine, it is subject to particular safety and quality standards[34]. Furthermore, some have noted that even in states and jurisdictions where CBD sale is illegal, lax enforcement of federal or state regulations allow for an easy ability to obtain CBD products[35].

The 2018 Farm Bill removed hemp's status as a Schedule 1 controlled substance which was a tremendous benefit for the cannabis market. By the Farm Bill's definition, 'hemp' became defined as any part or derivative of the *cannabis sativa* plant that contains less than 0.3% THC. So, by that definition, a hemp plant is not classified by its eventual use or by specific areas of the plant, but rather by a specific THC composition. However, the confusion becomes more apparent with CBD. In 2018, a CBD-based drug - Epidiolex® - was approved by the FDA for seizures. Because it was an FDA-approved drug, Epidiolex® could not fit under the Schedule 1 classification which in part claims that a drug in Schedule 1 has no medical use. Whereas Epidiolex® was approved as a drug, CBD – when used in Epidiolex® only – thereby 'gained' a medical use and was in turn moved to a Schedule V classification.

Once a CBD-based drug was reclassified as Schedule V, the CBD world effectively rejoiced at the news – but that was short-lived. It quickly became apparent that this reclassification was for FDA-approved drugs with very low THC levels. The confusion arose from the fact that, with the exception of Epidiolex®, CBD is 1) not FDA-approved, and 2) remains a marijuana derivative. Furthermore, the FDA has made it clear that it will pursue those who market cannabis-based products like CBD as 'therapeutic' in nature and will also pursue those who add cannabis products to food items or supplements used in interstate commerce[36].

So what does all of this mean to a patient? Basically, hemp-derived CBD has been made legal by the Farm Bill – as long as the portion of the cannabis plant used truly qualifies as hemp. The problem, as we will later discuss, is that there is very little CBD in the branches and stalks of the hemp plant. Therefore, it is important as a patient to understand the source and the chemical makeup of your CBD so as to stay on the right side of the law.

Why regulate?

Clearly, there is a change in attitudes as well as regulations specific to the outright banning of cannabis and cannabis-related products. The rationale behind these changes is multi-fold and has been said to include concerns that are both financial in nature and also geared toward addressing state incarceration rates[37, 38], yet also reflects changing attitudes toward the potential medical benefits of marijuana-based compounds[39, 40].

When looking around at all of the places to buy CBD that seemingly line the streets of certain states, it might make you wonder how they are regulated. Truth be told, none of them sell products that are approved by the FDA for safety or efficacy[41]. That's because, as we just discussed, CBD is not approved by the FDA – only Epidiolex® is approved as a CBD-based medicine. Because of the consequent lack of consistent standards related to CBD, state laws do not guarantee any sort of quality from the product itself[41]. Whereas CBD is derived from a plant that also has hallucinogenic qualities, any lack of regulation (or quality control) could easily subject a patient looking for anti-inflammatory effects in their CBD bottle to, for example, unwanted hallucinogenic or psychotropic effects if the THC levels are too high. Failing to regulate the source of CBD, such

31

as how CBD must be obtained from plants that have an upper-limit THC content, could ultimately subject you the patient to unintended effects of THC.

Conclusion

Without question, the cannabis plant has many diverse applications, some of which hold the potential to improve our health and well-being. As patients, we are always looking for a way to improve our health, and cannabis appears to hold the potential to influence a variety of ailments. Unfortunately for medical patients, cannabis comes with a wealth of restrictions specific to its use, harvest, and even how it is classified for agriculture or medicine. Despite changing attitudes along with lessened regulations towards cannabis use, there remains a convoluted path that must be followed in order to remain within the parameters of the law. The passage of the Farm Bill opened an important window into hemp use that has in turn created an explosion of interest in the cannabis industry, particularly regarding the use and potential benefits of CBD. Next, we'll change our focus temporarily from cannabis in order to outline the inner workings of the vestibular system. Given your interest in this book as a vestibular patient, I feel that it is relevant to orient you to how your balance and equilibrium are controlled by the body, so we'll outline those aspects in the next chapter. That, combined with your knowledge about CBD that will come in later chapters, will serve to allow you to have productive conversations with your medical provider specific to how CBD may influence these vestibular processes and potentially improve your health.

Chapter References

1.   Grigoryev, S., *Hemp (Cannabis sativa L.) genetic resources at the VIR: from the collection of seeds, through to the collection of sources, towards the collection of donors of traits. The history of cultivation of hemp in Russia.* 1998, Online publications, NI Vavilov Research Institute of Plant Industry ....

2.   Chandra, S., et al., *Cannabis cultivation: methodological issues for obtaining medical-grade product.* Epilepsy & Behavior, 2017. **70**: p. 302-312.

3.   Mechoulam, R., *The pharmacohistory of Cannabis sativa.* Cannabinoids as therapeutic agents, 1986: p. 1-19.

4.   Ligresti, A., L. De Petrocellis, and V. Di Marzo, *From phytocannabinoids to cannabinoid receptors and endocannabinoids: pleiotropic physiological and pathological roles through complex pharmacology.* Physiological reviews, 2016. **96**(4): p. 1593-1659.

5.   O'Shaughnessy, W.B., *Case of Tetanus, cured by a preparation of Hemp (the Cannabis indica).* Trans Med Phys Soc Bengal, 1839. **1838**: p. 462-469.

6.   Boire, R. and K. Feeney, *Medical Marijuana Law.* 2007: Ronin Publishing.

7.   Rovetto, L.J. and N.V. Aieta, *Supercritical carbon dioxide extraction of cannabinoids from Cannabis sativa L.* The Journal of Supercritical Fluids, 2017. **129**: p. 16-27.

8.   ElSohly, M.A. and D. Slade, *Chemical constituents of marijuana: the complex mixture of natural cannabinoids.* Life sciences, 2005. **78**(5): p. 539-548.

9.   Zou, S. and U. Kumar, *Cannabinoid receptors and the endocannabinoid system: signaling and function in the central nervous system.* International journal of molecular sciences, 2018. **19**(3): p. 833.

10.   Small, E., *Evolution and classification of Cannabis sativa (marijuana, hemp) in relation to human utilization.* The botanical review, 2015. **81**(3): p. 189-294.

11.   Johnson, R. *Defining "Industrial Hemp": A Fact Sheet.* in *LIBRARY OF CONGRESS WASHINGTON DC CONGRESSIONAL RESEARCH SERVICE.* 2017.

12.   Gertsch, J., R.G. Pertwee, and V. Di Marzo, *Phytocannabinoids beyond the Cannabis plant—do they exist?* British journal of pharmacology, 2010. **160**(3): p. 523-529.

13. Devane, W.A., et al., *Determination and characterization of a cannabinoid receptor in rat brain.* Molecular pharmacology, 1988. **34**(5): p. 605-613.

14. Russo, E.B., *Taming THC: potential cannabis synergy and phytocannabinoid-terpenoid entourage effects.* British journal of pharmacology, 2011. **163**(7): p. 1344-1364.

15. Izzo, A.A., et al., *Peripheral endocannabinoid dysregulation in obesity: relation to intestinal motility and energy processing induced by food deprivation and re-feeding.* British journal of pharmacology, 2009. **158**(2): p. 451-461.

16. Hemp Business Journal. *The U.S. Hemp Industry grows to $820mm in sales in 2017.* 2018.

17. Jagielski, D., *The Retail Market Will Make Up More Than 60% of CBD Sales in the U.S. by 2024,* in *The Motley Fool.* 2019.

18. United Nations, *World Drug Report 2015,* Office on Drugs and Crime, Editor. 2015.

19. Borchardt, D., *Marijuana sales totaled $6.7 billion in 2016.* Forbes. Retrieved from https://www. forbes. com/sites/debraborchardt/2017/01/03/marijuana-sales-totaled-6-7-billion-in-2016, 2017.

20. Sawler, J., et al., *The genetic structure of marijuana and hemp.* PloS one, 2015. **10**(8): p. e0133292.

21. Potter, D., *Growth and morphology of medicinal cannabis.* The medicinal uses of Cannabis and cannabinoids, 2004: p. 17-54.

22. Sirikantaramas, S., et al., *Tetrahydrocannabinolic acid synthase, the enzyme controlling marijuana psychoactivity, is secreted into the storage cavity of the glandular trichomes.* Plant and Cell Physiology, 2005. **46**(9): p. 1578-1582.

23. Sirikantaramas, S., et al., *The Gene Controlling Marijuana Psychoactivity MOLECULAR CLONING AND HETEROLOGOUS EXPRESSION OF Δ1-TETRAHYDROCANNABINOLIC ACID SYNTHASE FROM CANNABIS SATIVA L.* Journal of Biological Chemistry, 2004. **279**(38): p. 39767-39774.

24. Johnston, D. and N.A. Lewis, *Obama administration to stop raids on medical marijuana dispensers.* New York Times, 2009. **18**.

25. Hartig, H. and A. Geiger, *About six-in-ten Americans support marijuana legalization. Pew Research Center.* 2018.

26. Wallace, A. and J. Steffen, *Colorado Supreme Court: Employers can fire for off-duty pot use.* Denver Post, 2015.

27.   Network of Trial Law Firms. *In the Weeds: Marijuana Legalization & Employment Laws*. 2019.

28.   Pacula, R.L. and E.L. Sevigny, *Marijuana liberalizations policies: why we can't learn much from policy still in motion.* Journal of policy analysis and management:[the journal of the Association for Public Policy Analysis and Management], 2014. **33**(1): p. 212.

29.   National Conference of State Legislatures. *State Medical Marijuana Laws*. 2019.

30.   National Conference of State Legislatures. *Marijuana Overview*. 2019.

31.   VanDolah, H.J., B.A. Bauer, and K.F. Mauck. *Clinicians' guide to cannabidiol and hemp oils*. in *Mayo Clinic Proceedings*. 2019. Elsevier.

32.   United States Congress, *115 th Congress. December 2018.* Agriculture Improvement Act of 2018.

33.   Pacula, R.L. and R. Smart, *Medical marijuana and marijuana legalization.* Annual review of clinical psychology, 2017. **13**: p. 397-419.

34.   Food, U. and D. Administration, *FDA and Marijuana: Questions and Answers.* Page Last Updated, 2017. **8**: p. 15.

35.   Hazekamp, A., *The trouble with CBD oil.* Medical cannabis and cannabinoids, 2018. **1**(1): p. 65-72.

36.   United States Food and Drug Administration, *FDA warns 15 companies for illegally selling various products containing cannabidiol as agency details safety concerns*, in *Violations include marketing unapproved new human and animal drugs, selling CBD products as dietary supplements, and adding CBD to human, animal foods.* 2019.

37.   Raphael, S. and M.A. Stoll, *Why are so many Americans in prison?* 2013: Russell Sage Foundation.

38.   Caulkins, J.P., et al., *Considering marijuana legalization: Insights for Vermont and other jurisdictions.* 2015: Rand Corporation.

39.   Koppel, B.S., et al., *Systematic review: efficacy and safety of medical marijuana in selected neurologic disorders: report of the Guideline Development Subcommittee of the American Academy of Neurology.* Neurology, 2014. **82**(17): p. 1556-1563.

40.   Hill, K.P., *Medical marijuana for treatment of chronic pain and other medical and psychiatric problems: a clinical review.* Jama, 2015. **313**(24): p. 2474-2483.

41.   Mead, A., *The legal status of cannabis (marijuana) and cannabidiol (CBD) under US law.* Epilepsy & Behavior, 2017. **70**: p. 288-291.

Chapter 2 – The Vestibular System

W HILE IT MIGHT BE of interest to dive right into the intricacies of cannabis and its derivatives, I think it better that we first outline the underlying anatomy and physiology involved with the vestibular system. In doing so, it can help provide you a relevant background that can serve as a foundation for the endocannabinoid system. In using this chapter to understand the anatomy that is likely associated with many of the vestibular disorders, you will be able to later visualize the affected structures and also be able to differentiate many of the associated components of the inner ear. So while this chapter may seem somewhat like an anatomy book at times, its real purpose is to provide you a solid foundation specific to both the anatomy involved with the vestibular system itself as well as provide you an overview of those structures that can influence balance, dizziness, and vertigo.

The rationale for being all-inclusive with the anatomy of the ear is that when these balance-related structures are functioning incorrectly, we are left with what ends up being some of the symptoms of many vestibular disorders: imbalance, dizziness, and possibly a bit of vertigo. Therefore, this chapter will highlight not only the major components of our inner ear but will also outline how several of these structures are responsible for our ability to maintain balance and equilibrium.

Sections of the ear

Outer ear

The most noticeable component of what we commonly characterize as our 'ear' is the portion that we can see (Figure 2.1). This includes the large pinna as well as the ear canal that leads to the eardrum, which collectively makes up our outer ear. The function of the outer ear is largely limited to funneling sound into the eardrum, and as it is located well away from the inner ear structures, the outer ear is not considered to have any involvement with the symptoms associated with vestibular-based disorders.

Middle ear

The middle ear is the air-filled portion of the ear located behind the eardrum and housed within the temporal bone (Figure 2.1). This portion of the ear holds the three small bones – the malleus, stapes, and incus – that transfer sound from the eardrum to the inner ear. The most association you will likely have with the middle ear is when you suffer the effects of an ear infection. As the middle ear is really nothing more than a space within the temporal bone, it too has no real involvement with most vestibular disorders, but may play a role in dizziness or instability among patients who are afflicted temporarily with an inner-ear infection.

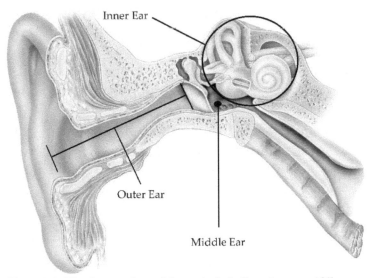

Figure 2.1. The three sections of the ear include the outer ear, middle ear, and inner ear. Issues involved with PPPD influence signals that are sent from the labyrinth portion of the inner ear

Inner ear

The inner ear is responsible for two major roles in our body. First, it detects and converts sound waves to neural impulses. In other words, it is responsible for our sense of hearing. While this is certainly no small feat, the inner ear is also responsible for the perception and interpretation of body positioning. This in turn makes the inner ear the site of both our main balance organ and our primary hearing organ.

Because of the intricate roles it has specific to hearing and motion detection, the inner ear is comprised of an array of highly sensitive structures. Unfortunately, the sensitivity of these structures also makes the inner ear quite susceptible to injury. Despite its small size, intricate structure, and dual responsibility for handling detection of both sound and motion, damage to the sensitive components of the inner ear can affect aspects that range from hearing to equilibrium. Furthermore, even minor disruptive events can trigger several symptoms such as motion sickness, vertigo, or nausea. Because of the high level of involvement of the inner ear structures in detecting sound and motion, the inner ear has been called one of the most intensively studied areas of vertebrate anatomy and physiology[1].

There are two main areas that make up the inner ear – the cochlea and the vestibular system. Together, these two structures make up what is known as the *labyrinth*. Despite what you often see in images of the inner ear, the labyrinth organs are

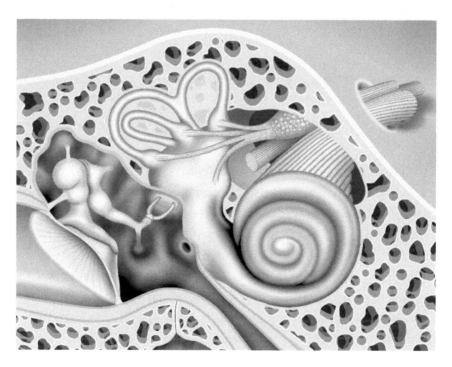

Figure 1.2. The labyrinth system does not consist of free-standing structures but rather a group of hollowed-out areas of the temporal bone that form a series of cavities and tunnels

not free-standing structures; rather, they are simply tunnels that exist deep within the temporal bone (Figure 2.2). These tunnels contain membranes that serve to contain the unique fluid (i.e. 'endolymph') contained within the labyrinth. As we will discuss, it is the movement of this fluid within the vestibular system that provides much of our ability to detect certain motions of the head.

The vestibular system

Although the inner ear isn't specifically implicated in all vestibular disorders (e.g. Mal de Debarquement syndrome), many of its components are thought to play a role in the associated symptoms of many disorders such as vertigo or constant dizziness. Therefore, we will next take a detailed look at the structure and function of these inner ear components thought to play a role in the symptoms associated with many vestibular disorders.

There are two primary systems at play within the inner ear (Figure 2.3). The first is the cochlea, a snail shaped organ designed to convert sound waves to electrical signals that can be interpreted by the brain as 'sound'. Within the cochlea are thousands of hair cells that are connected via nerves to the brain. These hair cells are bathed in potassium-rich fluid called endolymph. Vibrations from the eardrum are transmitted by way of the middle ear bones to the cochlea, where these vibrations are eventually detected by cochlear hair cells which then convert the vibrations into a neural signal by way of the organ of Corti. The hair cells of the cochlea are highly sensitive and are therefore subject to damage from a variety of causes such as loud noise, antibiotic medication, or certain diseases such as meningitis. Damage to cochlear hair cells is particularly unfortunate as they are unable to regenerate. Consequently, any cochlear hair cells damaged beyond repair permanently decrease the number of working hair cells.

While some vestibular disorders do have an association with hearing loss, not all are known to affect hearing. Furthermore, even within some conditions such as Ménière's disease, among two patients experiencing drop attacks it may occur that only one exhibits hearing deficits. Regardless, because its role is limited to hearing-based events, the cochlea is not directly involved in most of the detrimental effects that occur in conjunction with vestibular disorders. Therefore, the remainder of this chapter will focus predominantly on the vestibular system given its strong link to the symptoms that commonly occur in response to vestibular disorders.

In terms of an overall purpose, the vestibular system of the inner ear has a primary role of detecting motion of the head, along with serving to provide feedback specific to an individual's head position. It is known that structures of the vestibular system are involved in many vestibular-based disorders; therefore we will take a comprehensive look at the components of the vestibular system in order to outline how aspects such as unsteadiness or vertigo – both commonly associated with conditions such as Ménière's disease and vestibular migraine – may develop. To do this, we first need to detail the anatomy of our vestibular system as well as the physiology of how these structures work to provide feedback specific to our head's movement and position.

Vestibular anatomy

Five independent inner ear structures are involved in our ability to detect motion. The first two structures are housed within an organ termed the vestibule, a 3-5mm wide structure located between the cochlea and semicircular canals. The vestibule itself contains two very important components called the *saccule* and the *utricle* that are responsible for detecting motion that occurs in a linear direction (i.e. forward/backward, up/down, side-to-side). Activities such as running, walking,

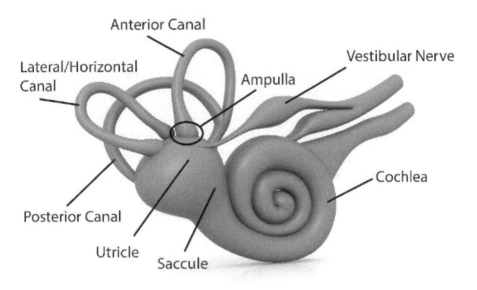

Figure 2.3. Vestibular anatomy consists of structures including the cochlea, the utricle and saccule contained within the vestibular, and the three semi-circular canals

standing up, or even riding in an elevator are detected by the saccule and the utricle, and as we will discuss, both structures have thousands of small crystals embedded within them to help detect inertia. It is this inertia and the resulting motion of the saccule and utricle that is then processed and interpreted by the brain as movement of the head. Because the saccule and utricle house these small crystals known as *otoliths*, the utricle and saccule are commonly known as the "otolith organs".

In addition to the saccule and utricle, the remainder of the vestibular portion of the inner ear is comprised of three tunnels called the anterior, horizontal, and posterior semicircular canals that form loops through the temporal bone. These canals detect circular motion, the kind generated when you shake your head 'yes' or 'no'. The semicircular canals also play a very important role in ensuring that our eyes can stay on a fixed spot or target even while our head is moving, through a process we will discuss later in this chapter known as the vestibulo-ocular reflex.

Without all of these structures functioning properly, our ability to maintain balance and have a normal equilibrium would be severely impaired. As we will outline, symptoms associated with many vestibular disorders such as benign paroxysmal positional vertigo (BPPV) or Ménière's disease appear to result from some improperly functioning component of the vestibular system in that either the system itself is not working or some aspect is excessively sensitive to motion. To help clarify how all of these components interact to work as a functioning unit, we will next take a look at the individual structures of the vestibular system along with outlining how they work to help us detect movement and maintain equilibrium.

Saccule

The saccule is a structure within the vestibule that is responsible for detecting vertical motion of the head (and with movement of the head typically comes movement of the body as well). For example, jumping up and down or riding in an elevator are activities that stimulate the motion sensors within the saccule. Inside the saccule is a structure called the *macula sacculi*, a vertically-oriented organ which houses a two- to three-millimeter area comprised of sensory hair cells responsible for detecting head motion. The ends of these hair cells extend horizontally into the middle of the vestibule and are covered by a gelatinous layer, over which is a fibrous structure called the otolithic membrane (Figure 2.4). This otolithic membrane is embedded with thousands of calcium-based crystals known by a variety of names including *statoconia, otoconia,* and the aforementioned *otolith.* For the purpose of this book we will use the term *otolith* to describe the crystals of the inner ear.

Because it is embedded with otoliths, the otolithic membrane is heavier than the material surrounding it.

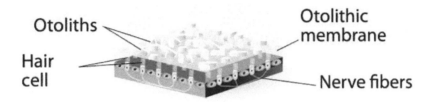

Figure 2.4 Otoliths embedded within the otolithic membrane activate hair cells in response to directional head motion (image is of the orientation of the macula utriculi)

Therefore, when the body moves somewhat quickly in a vertical plane such as occurs when jumping, gravity pulls the otoliths downward the same way as a leafy branch might bend when you swing it upward. The weight of the otoliths causes nerve cells that extend into the otolithic membrane to bend in response to the linear motion. This in turn triggers those hair cells to send a signal to the brain that is interpreted as vertical movement of the head.

Utricle

The utricle has an almost identical makeup as the saccule but has a slightly different orientation and function. The utricle is larger than the saccule and operates by detecting when the head moves in the horizontal plane. Such movements, which occur with forward, backward, or side-to-side motion of the head, happen with walking, running, or even riding in a car. Like the saccule, the utricle contains a macula called the *macula utriculi*. In contrast to the saccule's vertically-oriented macula, the macula utriculi is positioned horizontally and is embedded with hair cells that are oriented vertically. The mechanism by which the macula utriculi detects motion operates similarly to that of the macula sacculi in that the hair cells are covered with a gelatinous layer which is in turn overlaid with a gel-like membrane embedded with otoliths.

Similar to the vertical action within the saccule, when forward, backward, or side-to-side head motion occurs within the utricle, the inertia created from the force of the motion upon the embedded otoliths creates a sort of 'shearing' motion between the gelatinous layer and the otolithic membrane. This motion is then detected by the utricle's embedded nerve cells which in turn send a signal to the brain that gets interpreted as a specific horizontal movement of the head.

Semicircular Canals

In addition to the vestibule's saccule and utricle structures, there are three semicircular canals of the inner ear's labyrinth network that make up the remainder of the vestibular system. As mentioned earlier, the semicircular canals are not true bony structures themselves; rather, they exist as 'tunnels' or canals through the temporal bone. Thin membranes line the bone-encased semicircular canals and serve to contain the fluid known as endolymph that is found throughout the labyrinth system. Like each maculi of the utricle and saccule that detect linear movement, rotational or 'angular' motions of the head cause this endolymph to move within the canals – a process that we will discuss shortly. An example of angular motion would include turning the head side-to-side as if watching a tennis match. Because this movement does not generate enough inertia within the inner ear to act upon the saccule or utricle, the design of the semicircular canals allows them to detect this angular motion as the endolymph flows across specialized sensors within each canal. The brain then interprets the signal from these sensors to establish the direction of head movement.

There are three independent semicircular canals – the anterior, posterior, and horizontal canals. The arrangement of the three canals positions them at right angles to each other which in turn allows all head motions to be detected. This design can be imagined by thinking of a corner of a cube – each of the three sides of the cube represents a different plane of movement similar to how any angular movement of the head can be detected by one or more of the semicircular canals.

So how does movement of fluid within the semicircular canals actually result in the brain being able to detect the motion? It's quite a fascinating process (at least in my mind!), actually. Angular motion is detected due to endolymph passing over a specialized organ within each canal called the *cupula*. Movement of the head in an angular motion (i.e. shaking the head 'no', nodding the head, etc.) causes movement of endolymph, which in turn flows across hair cells that move in response to the flow of endolymph. These hair cells are located within the canal itself, at each end of the semicircular canal in a bulged-out area called the *ampulla* (see Figure 1.3). Hair cells within the ampulla contain the cupula, a gelatinous layer over the hair cells that extends across the width of the ampulla.

Let's look at this process in a little more detail. When a person moves his or her head, the endolymph moves within the semicircular canal in response to the head movement. As the fluid moves, it flows around the cupula (Figure 2.5). As the fluid

47

motion of the endolymph pushes against the cupula, the cupula bends in response to the fluid moving over it. This causes hair

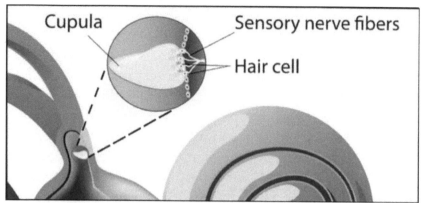

Figure 2.5. Near the end of each semicircular canal, the ampulla houses the sensitive cupula organ which is responsible for detecting movement of fluid within the respective semicircular canal

cells immediately under the cupula to also bend, the same way the aforementioned tree branch may bend if its leafy end were placed into flowing water. This bending of the hair cells sends a signal to the brain which is interpreted as motion appropriate to the direction of head movement.

These events occurring within the semicircular canals are important to understand, as they are largely thought to play a role in vertigo and dizziness. As far back as the 1960s, researchers believed that conditions such as BPPV – which triggers bouts of vertigo, nystagmus (rapid eye motion), and unsteadiness – resulted from otoliths pressing against the cupula within the semicircular canal[2]. This interference was suspected of increasing the cupula's sensitivity to motion, in turn generating the symptoms such as vertigo and nystagmus that are commonly associated with BPPV.

Vertigo and the vestibular system

The preceding portion of this chapter served to outline in detail much about the vestibular system as well as relevant cranial nerves that we rely on for daily function. My reasoning for going into such detail with each is two-fold. First, I want you to have an understanding of the complexity of the vestibular system, for as we have discussed, this system is quite intricate. Even a small disruption to the vestibular system can have a significant impact on several aspects of our life. The extent of this impact leads to the second reason I wanted to outline the vestibular system in depth – to help you understand the mechanisms involved in balance and vertigo that can arise as a result of many of the vestibular conditions, which we will discuss next.

Vertigo is the sensation of movement when in fact no movement is occurring. It is important to understand that vertigo is a symptom – not an actual medical condition; therefore, expecting a cure for vertigo is effectively the same as expecting a cure for pain. What is likely meant is that one expects a cure for what is *causing* the vertigo. Vertigo itself is largely thought to result from events occurring within the inner ear, and other medical conditions that trigger vertigo – such as BPPV – are known to originate from within the inner ear. Still, other vertigo-inducing conditions such as PPPD are not as clear cut and are thought to involve a complex interaction between the brain (i.e. 'central' type vertigo) and the inner ear (i.e. 'peripheral' vertigo).

As a patient of a vestibular-related condition it is important to understand that vertigo has several possible sources, and no one event or structure has been established as a primary cause for vertigo. Researchers have largely narrowed peripheral vertigo down to the semicircular canals, saccule, or utricle, while central vertigo is typically associated with either the brainstem or the vestibulocochlear nerve[3]. When functioning normally, the inner ear structures send signals to the brain in a coordinated pattern from the left and right ear. However, an imbalance of these vestibular inputs – such as can occur when one of our two vestibular systems is not performing correctly – leads to uncoordinated information being transmitted to the brain, in turn triggering events such as nystagmus (rapid and uncontrollable eye movement) or vertigo to occur. This imbalanced signal can occur due to disruption anywhere along the neural pathway that stretches from the vestibular-based sensors to the brain.

Again, there is no specific structure or area that triggers vertigo across all patients. Therefore, vertigo can arise from multiple causes and conditions. For example, patients experiencing migraine (i.e. a specific type of headache) sometimes experience vertigo similar to patients who have a disorder specific to the vestibule of the inner ear. Sometimes vertigo even originates outside of the skull, such as can occur in patients who experience vertigo that results from degrading intervertebral discs, a condition known as 'cervical vertigo'[4].

One confounding issue that medical professionals have in establishing vertigo is that patients often lump it in with dizziness. Both vertigo and dizziness are indeed similar in their effects given that each can make you as the patient feel unsteady. One recommended way to separate the two conditions is to determine whether you feel 'lightheaded' or whether you feel as though the world is spinning around you. Generally, a spinning sensation is more characteristic of vertigo, while lightheadedness is typically associated with dizziness[5].

To reiterate, the symptom of vertigo occurs when the patient reports that their world is spinning around them despite the fact that they are stationary. So what exactly causes this sensation? Physiologically speaking, the sensation of vertigo is largely thought to be due in part to a link between the inner ear and the eyes. While this may seem to be a somewhat odd link, the interconnection between our ears and eyes plays a vital role in our daily function even though we may not recognize it (until there is a problem!). To outline this role, we need to discuss the vestibulo-ocular reflex and how it coordinates the interaction between the ear and eye.

The vestibulo-ocular reflex (VOR)

Although our eyes have independent functions specific to providing our sense of vision, they are intimately connected with the inner ear. This interaction plays an important role in our ability to maintain balance as well as to maintain visual acuity when we are moving. To see how important your vision is for aiding in your balance, walk quickly from a bright room into a very dark one. You'll probably find that you are initially timid and a little bit unsteady, which will likely improve once your eyes adjust to the darkness. Similarly, jump up and down a few times and notice how your vision of the field around you remains quite clear and steady – a stark contrast from watching a video that was recorded on a camera you held while jumping. The ability to maintain this smooth field of vision even while engaged in strenuous activity such as jumping is because of the intricate link between the vestibular system and the eyes. In fact, this link has even been given a name – the 'vestibulo-ocular reflex' (VOR). We won't go deep into the details of how the VOR works, but we will next provide a general overview of the reflex as it relates to a few expected symptoms of several vestibular conditions.

The interconnection between your vestibular system and eyes is what allows you to maintain a smooth, non-jumpy field of vision while running or riding on a bumpy road. This happens because the vestibular system actually has some control over the muscles of the eyes through the VOR that allows the eyes to remain fixed on an object even though one's head position may be moving. This reflex has the task of trying to ensure that an image or object remains stable on an individual's retina in order to allow for proper processing by the brain[6]. Without the VOR, every time your head moves, you would consciously need to readjust your eye position back to the object you are looking at. With the VOR, however, your vestibular system is able to detect the speed of your head motion and automatically control the muscles of your eyes so that your gaze easily remains fixed on the object. This reflex also works well when driving, as every time you hit a bump or turn a corner your eyes are subconsciously controlled by the VOR rather than jumping all around while trying to manually reposition – which would certainly be a problem when operating a vehicle!

When the VOR is working correctly you don't even know that it's there. But when there is a disruption to the system – such as occurs in response to a vestibular-related disease such as vestibular migraine – the VOR becomes impaired and can lead to uncontrolled movements such as the aforementioned nystagmus or the spinning sensation associated with vertigo. Consequently, an affected patient is not able to coordinate their eye movements with the movements of their head. This can lead to jumpy or blurry vision, likely occurring most often when the head is moving or the patient's body is in motion. Another condition that can result is *oscillopsia,* a condition in which objects in the field of vision appear to float around even though they are in fact stationary, due in large part to the muscles of the eye being unable to keep the eye adequately fixed on one object.

Additional problems occur when a person with a faulty VOR tries to follow movement or read text on paper or a computer screen, an event known as *tracking*. With the VOR not allowing for smooth eye movement such as that required to follow a thrown ball or read printed text, it can be difficult for the patient to make the precise eye motions needed to properly intake visual information (i.e. identify and process the written words). Without a well-established link between our eyes and our ears, life would be much more difficult. But unfortunately, because of this link we must often pay the price of having visual disturbances such as vertigo or nystagmus any time our vestibular system is malfunctioning.

Conclusion

Clearly, the inner ear consists of highly intricate and complex structures that are vital for our normal function. Without a properly functioning vestibular system, our ability to maintain posture, recognize our movements, and sense positional changes can be extremely difficult. The intent of this chapter was to provide an overview of those structural components of the inner ear involved in many of the more common vestibular conditions. In addition, we touched on several unintended physiological processes (i.e. 'symptoms') that can occur in response to a vestibular disorder, such as vertigo. Understand that what we covered in this chapter is indeed quite generic in scope; there is in fact much, much more that we could discuss at a much deeper level. However, this is a book focused on introducing you to CBD rather than serving as a comprehensive guide to your vestibular system. Therefore, this chapter was written with the intent of providing you a very general introduction to how your vestibular system works. What you will hopefully find is that as you read through this book about the endocannabinoid system and CBD, the detailed information we discussed in this chapter becomes more relevant to you given that you now better understand the various anatomy and physiology of the inner ear. Now, we'll shift our focus again and outline the highly unique endocannabinoid system that exists within our bodies. We'll discuss the intricacies of how the endocannabinoid system works as well as describe how we are able to capture the power of the unique molecules of the cannabis plant to potentially improve our health and fight disease.

Chapter References

1. Ekdale, E.G., *Form and function of the mammalian inner ear.* Journal of anatomy, 2016. **228**(2): p. 324-337.
2. Schuknecht, H. and R. Ruby, *Cupulolithiasis,* in *Otophysiology.* 1973, Karger Publishers. p. 434-443.
3. Lawal, O. and D. Navaratnam, *Causes of Central Vertigo,* in *Diagnosis and Treatment of Vestibular Disorders.* 2019, Springer. p. 363-375.
4. Peng, B., *Cervical vertigo: historical reviews and advances.* World neurosurgery, 2018. **109**: p. 347-350.
5. Lee, A., *Diagnosing the cause of vertigo: a practical approach.* Hong Kong Med J, 2012. **18**(4): p. 327-32.
6. Glover, J.C., *Vestibular System,* in *Encyclopedia of Neuroscience,* L.R. Squire, Editor. 2004, Academic Press: Oxford. p. 127-132.

Chapter 3 – The Endocannabinoid System

We spent the last chapter discussing the intricacies of the vestibular system, of which many of us are afflicted on a daily basis. Now, we are going to shift our focus over to the endocannabinoid system in order to look at how our bodies utilize those cannabinoids once they are introduced into our system. In this chapter we will focus on the main aspects of the endocannabinoid system, emphasizing the inner workings of the specialized receptors, molecules, and enzymes that are involved in cannabinoid processing. Gaining an awareness of the endocannabinoid system will help you understand the intricate aspects of how our endocannabinoid system works and can provide you a unique insight specific to how cannabinoids affect you. Furthermore, the knowledge you pick up from this chapter can help you have educated and productive conversations with your health professional and can also serve to help you make more informed decisions about your CBD.

Much like how the last chapter on vestibular anatomy was not intended to sound like it was taken from an anatomy book, this chapter is not meant to come across as a biochemistry book. However, there may at times be some 'technical jargon' spread throughout this chapter that makes it appear as such. Rest assured that there is no intent on my part as the author to confuse you with biochemical concepts; rather, my intent is to help you understand how the body utilizes cannabinoids such as CBD and how they work to exert their beneficial effects. Understanding these processes has to involve a bit of discussion specific to anatomy and physiology, but I've worked to try to get the information condensed into a format that is relatable for everyone. In understanding the endocannabinoid system better, it will also serve to provide you a better grasp of the upcoming chapter that looks specifically at cannabidiol.

Background of the endocannabinoid system

At present, over 550 compounds are known to exist in *cannabis sativa*, including 113 phytocannabinoids as well as 120 chemicals known as terpenes that influence the fragrance associated with cannabis[1]. Given the compound-dense nature of the cannabis plant, our relative lack of understanding of the plant holds immense promise for the future, particularly in the area of medical therapies. While we have made significant progress in our knowledge about cannabis, when you combine that with the fact that we don't yet understand the underlying purpose of the endocannabinoid system, it suggests a wealth of promise for future research.

Cannabinoids have been a key part of living organisms for a very, very long time. In fact, the discovery of cannabinoids within a type of fungus has led researchers to suspect that cannabinoids have been around for over 150 million years[2]. This estimate indicates that cannabinoids have been around even longer than the actual cannabis plant[2].

While the origins of cannabinoids appear to have a defined path in history, the relatively brief history of our understanding of the endocannabinoid system has left science somewhat puzzled as to just what it is designed to do. Nature has a pretty good track record of revealing that if something exists, it tends to have an underlying purpose or function. And holding true with that belief, most scientists will agree that the endocannabinoid system likely has some specific purpose. The frustration lies in the fact that we just haven't figured that purpose out yet.

Our current understanding of the endocannabinoid system came about through a series of steps that originated with trying to outline the various medical benefits of cannabis. As we discussed earlier, once THC was isolated from cannabis a search began in order to determine how THC exerted its effects on our body. This in turn led to the eventual discovery of cannabinoid receptors, followed by the discovery of those compounds – later named 'cannabinoids' – which could bind to those cannabinoid receptors. Work then focused on trying to understand the cannabinoids including their purpose as well as the mechanism for how they exert their effects. With only a couple of decades of focused work so far, there is much, much more to learn about understanding the potential power of the endocannabinoid system. As such, research is ongoing, trying to reveal key insights that will not only help us understand cannabinoids better but potentially provide us with preventative measures and, hopefully, potential cures.

The endocannabinoid system is considered to be critical for maintaining homeostasis (i.e. a stable environment) and human health[3]. Given the widespread distribution of endocannabinoid receptors in our body including several essential areas such as the cardiovascular system, revealing the purpose and role of the endocannabinoid system could ultimately have immense health implications. Scientists have long suspected that the endocannabinoid system plays an extensive role through interaction with several body processes including pain, appetite, mood, memory, and immunity, among others, and further research will help reveal the underlying potential that CBD may have.

Endocannabinoids

From a structural standpoint, endogenous cannabinoids are, at their basic level, fats that are capable of binding to specific cannabinoid receptors[4]. Similar to the process involved with all receptors in our body, once a cannabinoid binds to its receptor, it initiates a chemical signaling process that generates an effect (e.g. release of signaling molecules, halting continued release of molecules, etc.) that in turn triggers a particular outcome in the body (e.g. movement, pain, hormone release, etc.). The extent to which cannabinoids can influence or in some cases prevent these processes is ultimately what determines their degree of effectiveness.

When needed, certain endocannabinoids such as anandamide and 2-arachidonoylglycerol are produced in a process that starts with the release of specific components from the cell membrane such as arachidonic acid. These components are then reorganized through enzymatic action into their functional endocannabinoid structure for immediate use[4]. This process of immediate synthesis and use of endocannabinoids differs substantially from how other chemical signaling molecules in the body operate[5]. For example, neurotransmitters such as acetylcholine are synthesized by the body and then stored near their site of action at the neural synapse (i.e. nerve ending) where they are released upon activation of the nerve.

Phytocannabinoids

Research has shown that the cannabis plant has developed a wealth of cannabinoid structures as it has evolved. Genetic analysis has revealed that phytocannabinoid content of cannabis can differ significantly from other plants – even within the same strain of cannabis plant. Typically, the quantity of various phytocannabinoids is dependent upon the genetic makeup of the plant and as the plant ages, more cannabinoids that were created as an inactive version become biologically activated[6]. However, a genetic determination does not always hold true for cannabinoids. Even within Californian medical cannabis strains, the amount of cannabinoid can vary widely; therefore, the particular strain of plant should not be relied on as an indicator of the amount of phytocannabinoids present[7].

Whereas endocannabinoids are generated via components of the cell membrane, phytocannabinoids are synthesized first as an acidic 'pre-phytocannabinoid' that is then decarboxylated to form the final cannabinoid[8]. Therefore, CBD itself is not synthesized within cannabis in its end form; rather, it is developed within the plant as cannabidiolic acid. Later, it is converted chemically to CBD through factors such as age or heat[9].

It's not just a genetic factor that can result in phytocannabinoid variations, though. Aspects such as cultivation and storage techniques and even the plant's age upon harvest can influence their phytocannabinoid content[10]. For example, THC degrades to a molecule known as cannabinol as it ages in storage[10], indicating that the ratio of THC:cannabinol can be used as an indicator of the age of stored cannabis. Consequently, the potency of cannabis has been said to be represented by the total cannabinoid content[6]. Accordingly, it has been suggested that the actual cannabis as well as terpene content of a particular strain be made available for patients in order for them to evaluate the actual content[11].

Cannabinoid receptors

Receptors exist everywhere throughout the body and serve as 'receivers' of chemical messages sent by the body. Structurally speaking, receptors are small proteins embedded within the membrane of individual cells. Because each receptor has a unique structure, receptors can only bind with molecules that correspond to the specific structure of a receptor. In a broader sense, receptors can bind only to specific molecules in much the same way that locks can only be opened by a particular key. This specialized binding is vital, as the function of the entire body is largely dependent upon the action of receptors and their binding molecules. As we will show, at least one type of receptor in the endocannabinoid system operates using a mechanism quite unique from other receptors of the body.

The CB1 receptor

Within the endocannabinoid system, receptors exist in two types – cannabinoid receptor type-1 (CB1) and type-2 (CB2). The CB1 receptor is predominantly found throughout the central nervous system (i.e. brain and spinal cord). Interestingly, CB1 is found in high concentrations within particular areas of the brain including the basal ganglia – a section of the brain involved in control of physical movement – as well as in the cerebellum, hippocampus, and cerebral cortex areas that are responsible for not only control of movement but also memory and learning[5]. Of particular interest was the discovery that the CB1 receptor exists within all areas of the brain related to the processing of pain[12]. Although the CB1 receptor is primarily located within the central nervous system, it can also be found at low levels in other tissue such as the liver, muscle, heart, lung, and even sperm cells[5].

The CB1 receptor is considered the most common *metabotropic* (i.e. requires an additional physiological process to function) receptor in our brain[11]. Functionally speaking, the CB1 receptor is classified as a *retrograde messenger*. This designation means that unlike most receptors in the body that cause actions to happen further down a signaling pathway, CB1 receptors work somewhat 'backwards' by causing an inhibition of events that occur earlier in the signaling process (Figure 3.1).

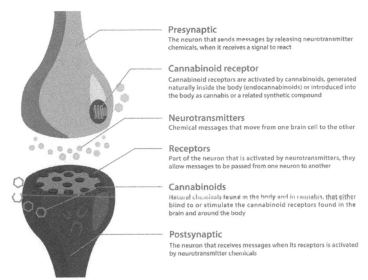

Presynaptic
The neuron that sends messages by releasing neurotransmitter chemicals, when it receives a signal to react

Cannabinoid receptor
Cannabinoid receptors are activated by cannabinoids, generated naturally inside the body (endocannabinoids) or introduced into the body as cannabis or a related synthetic compound

Neurotransmitters
Chemical messages that move from one brain cell to the other

Receptors
Part of the neuron that is activated by neurotransmitters, they allow messages to be passed from one neuron to another

Cannabinoids
Natural chemicals found in the body and in cannabis, that either blind to or stimulate the cannabinoid receptors found in the brain and around the body

Postsynaptic
The neuron that receives messages when its receptors is activated by neurotransmitter chemicals

Figure 2.1. Endocannabinoid receptors embedded in the pre-synaptic neuron detect cannabinoids released from the post-synaptic neuron, whereas neurotransmitters are released from the pre-synaptic neuron and detected by the post-synaptic neuron

To outline the difference between CB1 receptors and traditional receptors, let's look at an example. At typical nerve endings a neurotransmitter such as acetylcholine is released from a pre-synapse and diffuses to the post-synapse where it binds to its receptor. Once the signaling molecule binds to its receptor, that receptor is activated to initiate a subsequent chemical-based event called a *signal transduction cascade* that eventually leads to some major event in the body (e.g. muscle contraction, pain inhibition, etc.). With retrograde signaling such as found with CB1 receptors, however, endocannabinoids such as 2-arachidonoylglycerol (2-AG) and anandamide are released at the post-synapse and travel 'backward' to the pre-synapse where they bind to CB1 receptors. The CB1 receptor then undergoes its own signal transduction cascade to inhibit any additional pre-synapse transmitter release[5]. Chemically speaking, the actions that endocannabinoids ultimately trigger include inhibition of adenylate cyclase enzyme activity as well as decreasing cyclic adenosine monophosphate (cAMP) levels[13]. These collective actions serve to inhibit further neurotransmitter release, which in effect means that endocannabinoids serve to terminate certain physiological events due to the inhibitory action of their receptors (as opposed to *excitatory* action which would cause a receptor to initiate a physiological event). As research continues, this endocannabinoid signaling mechanism of blocking subsequent neurotransmitter release could have major implications as to understanding the endocannabinoid response, depending on what the ultimate physiological outcome of the particular neurotransmitter's release is such as tinnitus, pain, nausea, etc.

The CB1 receptor's location in the brain helps explain the expected response of euphoria (i.e. "high") that THC users experience, as CB1 is a main receptor for THC[13]. Like THC, anandamide – the first-discovered cannabinoid in humans – has a major influence on brain functioning. Interestingly, THC serves as a phytocannabinoid substitute for anandamide[14]. It is also noteworthy that of all the phytocannabinoids that interact with the CB1 receptor, THC is the strongest[15].

The CB2 receptor

Unlike CB1 receptors and their well-documented retrograde messaging system, not much is currently known about how CB2 receptors work[5]. CB2 receptors are found in small amounts within the brain's cerebellum and also in the brain stem[16], but there is also a widespread presence of CB2 among the immune (e.g. spleen), reproductive, and cardiovascular cells of the body[17] as well as within muscle, liver, intestinal, and fat tissue[18]. Despite this widespread presence of CB2 receptors, endocannabinoids actually have a greater general affinity for the CB1 receptor than the CB2 receptor[19].

While CB2's underlying function remains somewhat murky compared to the CB1 receptor, it is suspected that the CB2 receptor plays a role in helping to regulate inflammation within the liver. This in turn suggests an overriding role for the CB2 receptor as a protective agent for the body[20]. In addition, bone remodeling is suspected to be controlled in part by the action of CB2 receptors[21], and there appears to be some interplay between CB2 receptors and disease states. For example, the brain is known to be quite low in CB2 receptors yet certain diseases such as Alzheimer's and Huntington's disease have been shown to significantly elevate the level of CB2 receptors[22]. Furthermore, it is thought that CB2 may be involved in controlling CNS-associated diseases such as depression and substance abuse. This association between CB2 receptors and disease may explain the purported effects that endocannabinoids such as CBD can have on neurological-based conditions including epilepsy, seizure, Parkinson's, multiple sclerosis, and Alzheimer's, among others[8].

As of 2019 over 113 phytocannabinoids have been discovered, including CBD, *cannabinol*, and *cannabigerol*, among others. Depending on when you ultimately read this book, there may well be many more than the 113 currently-recognized cannabinoids, which would indicate that ongoing research has continued to identify additional components of cannabis. As more cannabinoids are identified, additional and potentially promising benefits specific to the action of those cannabinoids may be revealed. Perhaps hidden in a cannabinoid is an effective treatment for tinnitus, or vestibular migraine, or other devastating vestibular condition. Such efforts to find more potentially beneficial aspects of cannabis require research, which ultimately requires funding. As a patient of any medical disorder, the hope remains that funding can be directed towards appropriate research projects aimed at further revealing key aspects of the many cannabinoids tucked away inside the mysterious cannabis plant.

Terpenes

Although we are ultimately focusing on cannabinoids as a key component of the endocannabinoid system, we should commit some attention toward what are known as *terpenes*, a group of well over 100 different phytochemicals within the cannabis plant[23]. Terpenes exist within the cannabis plant's resin in a variety of forms including monoterpenes, diterpenes, and triterpenes, and are largely responsible for cannabis' unique aromatic properties. It is suspected, however, that terpenes do more than just provide cannabis' unique aroma, as some researchers suspect that terpenes may interact with cannabinoids to produce therapeutic effects.

Because of their structure, terpenes have the freedom to cross the blood-brain barrier and interact directly with brain tissue. There is evidence that they can influence other cannabis derivatives such as cannabinoids[24]. However, recent research indicates that several terpenes do not activate CB1 or CB2 receptors as endocannabinoids do[25], nor do terpenes influence the action of THC as CBD is capable of doing. Despite this apparent lack of interaction, research is focusing on therapies designed to capture the *combined* effect of cannabinoids and terpenes. Of particular interest, given terpene's ability to reach the brain, are therapies utilizing a combination of cannabinoids and terpenes in a 'synergistic' approach to target conditions such as sleeping disorders and social anxiety[26]. Evidence for a potential synergistic benefit in cannabis use was outlined in one study in mice that looked at the effect of a pure CBD preparation versus an extract of *cannabis sativa* that had the same concentration of CBD[27]. It was found that pure CBD had a minimal effect on colitis in those mice while the extract had a much greater effect. While this single study was not conclusive of any synergistic effect, such findings lend evidence to a potential benefit in providing CBD with other substances such as additional cannabinoids or terpenes.

The concept of synergism has been investigated at length in the cannabis world. The medical benefits reported amongst the many cannabis varieties have been suggested to occur at least in part through specific interactions between cannabinoids and terpenes in what has been termed an 'entourage effect'[26]. However, the potential for an interactive approach may come with some resistance. One author highlighted an interesting point regarding patients and their acceptance of such synergism in their medications[14]. Specifically, it was discussed that such a synergistic effect resulting from cannabis therapy can be difficult for patients in the United States to accept. This apprehension may in part be due to an over-reliance on pharmaceutical intervention amongst patients in developed nations such as the U.S. In effect, the researcher suggested that patients tend to expect 'single-pill' treatments which in turn cause us to be hesitant to expect benefits from plant-based therapies[14]. Consequently, the use of a cannabis-based preparation designed to utilize an 'entourage effect' may be met with a bit of hesitation on the part of the patient, in turn reducing the opportunity for the potential synergistic effects from a cannabinoid/terpene interaction capable of improving the therapeutic treatment effects or potentially inhibiting certain unfavorable physiological events such as pain.

It's worth noting that in addition to cannabinoids, medical marijuana is often pointed out as a potentially synergistic treatment[28]. The potential rationale for any existing synergism has not been revealed, but the evidence outlines that synergism could be a key aspect of a potential link between cannabinoids and terpenes or even between individual cannabinoid types that exist in cannabis extract but not in products such as pure CBD.

Despite evidence of no interaction specifically with CB1 or CB2 receptors, it remains possible that terpenes exert their effects using a mechanism that is similar to cannabinoids or perhaps different altogether. Given the vast number of terpenes present in cannabis combined with many as-yet unexplained effects from cannabinoids, the possibility of a synergistic effect between these substances warrants ongoing research.

A perplexing system

Oddly enough, despite the breadth of the endocannabinoid system's presence within our body, understanding the true purpose or function of the system remains perplexing for scientists. As we outlined earlier, endocannabinoids play a role in suppressing subsequent neurotransmitter release; however, the question remains as to *why* the body has developed this function. For example, healthy mice have had their endocannabinoid receptors genetically removed from their peripheral (non-brain) organs yet they develop no evident biological consequence[29]. Removing our cardiovascular or endocrine system is not possible due to the obvious fatal effects, but the question remains as to why the body might have developed a system such as the endocannabinoid system if it can also apparently survive without it. The expanse of the endocannabinoid system to practically all of our body's tissues suggests a definite purpose for its inclusion, but it's more likely that we just haven't yet been able to figure out why it is there, nor exactly how it functions.

From a medical sense, the endocannabinoid system has become a major point of interest for pharmaceutical research given its extensive role in the body. For example, substances that bind to CB1 and CB2 receptors have been used to help suppress nausea, to stimulate appetite, and as pain relievers for some diseases[11]. Unfortunately, some synthetic (i.e. 'man-made') forms of CB1-based endocannabinoids have been shown to have significant adverse effects that ultimately prevented further investigation[30]. Still, given the potential benefits of cannabinoid use, there are ongoing efforts to outline ways to suppress these unfortunate side effects, including trying to develop CB2 receptor-based drugs that can have similar effects as when binding to CB1 receptors[11].

Medical effects of cannabinoids

Thus far we have spent our time outlining how cannabinoids and related chemicals work within the body. Now, let's focus our attention toward exploring the effects that cannabinoids can have on the body which in turn helps explain their purpose. For one, it has long been known that cannabis use can influence the digestive system. Research has shown conclusively that endocannabinoids can promote appetite through interaction with CB1, and removing CB1 receptors in mice resulted in a sharp decrease in appetite[31]. Similarly, THC has been shown to help regulate the motility of food through the gut, as oral ingestion of THC slowed the movement of food through the intestines[32]. Along these same lines of intestinal interaction, research has shown that a change in the acidity (i.e. pH level) of the gut can cause activation of cannabinoid receptors[29]. Such information could be valuable for patients with intestinal issues such as Crohn's disease or even simple diarrhea, though much work remains to be done in this area.

Diet may also play a role in influencing the activity of the endocannabinoid system. In fact, evidence suggests that hunger itself may be controlled in part through activation of CB1 receptors in the intestine[33]. Diet composition may affect endocannabinoids, as mice fed a high-fat diet showed decreased movement of food through the small intestine while also exhibiting decreased anandamide levels in conjunction with significantly higher 2-AG levels[34]. In related research, several studies have reported that dietary fat intake is partially driven by endocannabinoid signaling within the intestines[35].

Obesity has been shown to increase the number of CB1 and CB2 receptors in the body[29]. This is important, given that CB1 receptor activation increases our intake of food and also influences the metabolism rate of other tissues[29]. This evidence might seem to infer that chronic marijuana users would be more susceptible to obesity, but strangely enough that is not the case. In fact, researchers suggest that chronic marijuana use may actually stimulate the body to decrease the amount of CB1 receptors[29], perhaps as a protective mechanism against a constant caloric intake.

Conclusion

In looking across the range of evidence that exists throughout the medical literature, there's little doubt that the endocannabinoid system plays a key role in our health. From unique signaling mechanisms to potentially synergistic effects, the apparent uniqueness of the endocannabinoid system reveals that we have much to learn in order to capture its potential benefits. Whereas the endocannabinoid system is quite new in terms of its discovery, the potential for additional findings specific to its purpose and inner workings is certainly promising. Furthermore, the fact that phytocannabinoid discovery continues to occur – along with the possibility for discovering an interaction between cannabinoids and terpenes – indicates that there is much to be optimistic about specific to the endocannabinoid system. In the next chapter we'll turn our attention from the endocannabinoid system itself to this book's cannabinoid of interest – cannabidiol – in order to outline its characteristics as well as the many health benefits that it may bring.

Chapter References

1.   Calvi, L., et al., *Comprehensive quality evaluation of medical Cannabis sativa L. inflorescence and macerated oils based on HS-SPME coupled to GC–MS and LC-HRMS (q-exactive orbitrap®) approach.* Journal of pharmaceutical and biomedical analysis, 2018. **150**: p. 208-219.
2.   Pacioni, G., et al., *Truffles contain endocannabinoid metabolic enzymes and anandamide.* Phytochemistry, 2015. **110**: p. 104-110.
3.   Cristino, L., T. Becker, and V. Di Marzo, *Endocannabinoids and energy homeostasis: an update.* Biofactors, 2014. **40**(4): p. 389-397.
4.   Lu, H.-C. and K. Mackie, *An introduction to the endogenous cannabinoid system.* Biological psychiatry, 2016. **79**(7): p. 516-525.
5.   Lu, D. and D. Potter, *Cannabinoids and the cannabinoid receptors: An overview*, in *Handbook of Cannabis and Related Pathologies.* 2017, Elsevier. p. 553-563.
6.   Hädener, M., S. König, and W. Weinmann, *Quantitative determination of CBD and THC and their acid precursors in confiscated cannabis samples by HPLC-DAD.* Forensic science international, 2019. **299**: p. 142-150.
7.   Elzinga, S., et al., *Cannabinoids and terpenes as chemotaxonomic markers in cannabis.* Natural Products Chemistry & Research, 2015. **2015**.
8.   Marcu, J.P., *An overview of major and minor phytocannabinoids*, in *Neuropathology of drug addictions and substance misuse.* 2016, Elsevier. p. 672-678.
9.   Citti, C., et al., *Analysis of cannabinoids in commercial hemp seed oil and decarboxylation kinetics studies of cannabidiolic acid (CBDA).* Journal of pharmaceutical and biomedical analysis, 2018. **149**: p. 532-540.
10.   Potter, D.J., *A review of the cultivation and processing of cannabis (Cannabis sativa L.) for production of prescription medicines in the UK.* Drug testing and analysis, 2014. **6**(1-2): p. 31-38.
11.   Aizpurua-Olaizola, O., et al., *Targeting the endocannabinoid system: future therapeutic strategies.* Drug discovery today, 2017. **22**(1): p. 105-110.

12. Starowicz, K. and D.P. Finn, *Cannabinoids and pain: sites and mechanisms of action*, in *Advances in Pharmacology*. 2017, Elsevier. p. 437-475.

13. Pertwee, R., *The diverse CB1 and CB2 receptor pharmacology of three plant cannabinoids: Δ9-tetrahydrocannabinol, cannabidiol and Δ9-tetrahydrocannabivarin.* British journal of pharmacology, 2008. **153**(2): p. 199-215.

14. Small, E., *Evolution and classification of Cannabis sativa (marijuana, hemp) in relation to human utilization.* The botanical review, 2015. **81**(3): p. 189-294.

15. Gertsch, J., R.G. Pertwee, and V. Di Marzo, *Phytocannabinoids beyond the Cannabis plant—do they exist?* British journal of pharmacology, 2010. **160**(3): p. 523-529.

16. Piomelli, D., *The molecular logic of endocannabinoid signalling.* Nature Reviews Neuroscience, 2003. **4**(11): p. 873.

17. Derbenev, A.V., T.C. Stuart, and B.N. Smith, *Cannabinoids suppress synaptic input to neurones of the rat dorsal motor nucleus of the vagus nerve.* The Journal of physiology, 2004. **559**(3): p. 923-938.

18. García-Bueno, B. and J.R. Caso, *Cannabis, Cannabinoid Receptors, and Stress-Induced Excitotoxicity*, in *Neuropathology of Drug Addictions and Substance Misuse*. 2016, Elsevier. p. 731-737.

19. Tabrizi, M.A. and P. Baraldi, *Chemistry of Cannabinoid Receptor Agonists*, in *Handbook of Cannabis and Related Pathologies*. 2017, Elsevier. p. 592-605.

20. Mallat, A., et al., *The endocannabinoid system as a key mediator during liver diseases: new insights and therapeutic openings.* British journal of pharmacology, 2011. **163**(7): p. 1432-1440.

21. Tam, J., et al., *Involvement of neuronal cannabinoid receptor CB1 in regulation of bone mass and bone remodeling.* Molecular pharmacology, 2006. **70**(3): p. 786-792.

22. Palazuelos, J., et al., *Microglial CB2 cannabinoid receptors are neuroprotective in Huntington's disease excitotoxicity.* Brain, 2009. **132**(11): p. 3152-3164.

23. Brenneisen, R., *Chemistry and analysis of phytocannabinoids and other Cannabis constituents*, in *Marijuana and the Cannabinoids*. 2007, Springer. p. 17-49.

24. Aizpurua-Olaizola, O., et al., *Evolution of the cannabinoid and terpene content during the growth of Cannabis sativa plants from different chemotypes.* Journal of natural products, 2016. **79**(2): p. 324-331.

25.   Santiago, M.J., et al., *Absence of entourage: Terpenoids commonly found in Cannabis sativa do not modulate the functional activity of Δ9-THC at human CB1 and CB2 receptors.* bioRxiv, 2019: p. 569079.

26.   Russo, E.B., *Taming THC: potential cannabis synergy and phytocannabinoid-terpenoid entourage effects.* British journal of pharmacology, 2011. **163**(7): p. 1344-1364.

27.   Pagano, E., et al., *An orally active Cannabis extract with high content in cannabidiol attenuates chemically-induced intestinal inflammation and hypermotility in the mouse.* Frontiers in pharmacology, 2016. **7**: p. 341.

28.   Russo, E.B. and J.M. McPartland, *Cannabis is more than simply Δ 9-tetrahydrocannabinol.* Psychopharmacology, 2003. **165**(4): p. 431-432.

29.   Scudellari, M. *Your body is teeming with weed receptors.* 2017; Available from: https://www.the-scientist.com/features/your-body-is-teeming-with-weed-receptors-31233.

30.   Kreitzer, F.R. and N. Stella, *The therapeutic potential of novel cannabinoid receptors.* Pharmacology & therapeutics, 2009. **122**(2): p. 83-96.

31.   Di Marzo, V., et al., *Leptin-regulated endocannabinoids are involved in maintaining food intake.* Nature, 2001. **410**(6830): p. 822.

32.   Chesher, G., et al., *The effect of cannabinoids on intestinal motility and their antinociceptive effect in mice.* British journal of pharmacology, 1973. **49**(4): p. 588-594.

33.   DiPatrizio, N.V., et al., *Fasting stimulates 2-AG biosynthesis in the small intestine: role of cholinergic pathways.* American Journal of Physiology-Regulatory, Integrative and Comparative Physiology, 2015. **309**(8): p. R805-R813.

34.   Izzo, A.A., et al., *Peripheral endocannabinoid dysregulation in obesity: relation to intestinal motility and energy processing induced by food deprivation and re-feeding.* British journal of pharmacology, 2009. **158**(2): p. 451-461.

35.   DiPatrizio, N.V., et al., *Endocannabinoid signal in the gut controls dietary fat intake.* Proceedings of the National Academy of Sciences, 2011. **108**(31): p. 12904-12908.

Chapter 4 – Cannabidiol

And now we have reached the topic of particular interest for so many vestibular patients - cannabidiol. Given the relative lack of a clear understanding that we currently have regarding CBD, we are caught in that informational vacuum of trying to gain enough evidence to determine whether CBD is a figurative 'godsend' or whether it will turn out to be nothing more than a passing fad. Until we have definitive answers that can be attained through quality research, we have to remain focused on what we've learned up to this point and take advantage of those apparent beneficial effects that surround this potential 'wonder molecule'. In this chapter, we'll focus on CBD specifically – what it is, purported safety, extraction techniques, and how it is used to help improve health and specific medical conditions. Topics from this chapter can provide you as a medical patient the most pertinent information specific to helping you decide whether cannabidiol is a viable treatment for your vestibular condition.

The basics of CBD

As discussed earlier, cannabidiol, or "CBD", is a phytocannabinoid that is the main non-psychoactive cannabinoid of the *cannabis sativa* plant. First discovered in its pure form after extraction from Mexican marijuana in 1940[1], CBD's chemical structure was later determined in 1963[2]. CBD comprises approximately 40% of cannabis extract, though actual CBD concentration within the cannabis plant is much less[3]. CBD is not actually the substance's natural form; rather, its cannabidiolic acid structure must be decarboxylated (through light, heat, or the aging process) which in turn produces CBD[4]. In addition to its role while in its active form, CBD also serves as a precursor of THC[5].

Despite a poor ability to bind to the CB1 receptor, CBD is somewhat unique in that when present in low levels it can inhibit the action of CB1 receptors[6]. In addition to its influence on CB1 and CB2 receptors, CBD has been shown to influence molecular signaling pathways involving 5-HT1A, GPR55, GPR18, and TRPV1 receptors among others[7]. For example, recent research has found that CBD influences the activity of 5HT(1A) receptors of the brain[8]. This finding could have significant implications as 5HT(1A) receptors inhibit 5-Hydroxytryptamine (5-HT)[9], a molecule better known by its common name 'serotonin'. Serotonin is a chemical used to facilitate communication between nerves but also influences psychological disorders such as anxiety and depression.

CBD has been grouped into a variety of uses including anti-emetic, anti-psychotic, anxiolytic (i.e. anxiety reducer), and anti-inflammatory[10]. While these effects have been demonstrated to some degree within the research, it has long been known that CBD – and to a lesser degree THC – have the ability to influence the formation of anti-inflammatory agents. Anti-inflammatory agents (e.g. 'eicosanoids') are formed from arachidonic acid that is contained within the cell membrane. CBD – and to a lesser degree THC – have been shown to trigger release of arachidonic acid from the cell membrane in some cells[11]. And in a related event, the type of anti-inflammatory produced (i.e. cyclo-oxygenase vs. lipoxygenase) has been shown to be dependent upon the presence of cannabinoids[12].

Market presence of CBD

Sales of CBD reached nearly $238 million in 2018, a 57% increase over the previous year[13]. Comparably speaking, with growing medical-based interest along with lessened regulations from the 2018 Farm Bill it is reasonable to expect continued growth in sales, perhaps even exponentially, with one projection predicting 107% annual growth in CBD sales through 2023[14]. Research interest has paralleled the growth in sales, as from 1999-2002 there were only 50 publications using the word cannabidiol while from 2008-2014 there were well over 1200[12]. Part of this recent research surge has been suggested to be due to the fact that THC received the majority of cannabinoid interest in years past, perhaps due to a belief that THC was initially thought to be the active component of cannabis as a result of its psychotropic potential[12]. One could assume that due to the focus on the therapeutic potential for THC, CBD was relegated to somewhat of an afterthought.

Defining the cannabidiol user

A variety of surveys and research studies exist specific to the typical user profile of CBD, but it is difficult to differentiate user data that was compiled with no scientific sampling procedures versus those which tried to get a valid cross-sectional sample of users. One Gallup poll from 2019 reported that 14% of Americans use CBD, indicating that a significant portion of the population has recognized the potential benefits of CBD[15]. A separate study provided a bit more insight into

CBD users, reporting that the predominant characteristics of CBD users include being a millennial (i.e. born 1981-1996), of the male gender, and possessing a college education[16]. Nearly half of males reported using CBD daily, while only around 3 in 10 female respondents indicated daily use. Millennial patients reported taking CBD more for anxiety and general health while "Gen X" users (those born between 1965 and 1980) took it more for joint and muscle pain. Interestingly, while over half of the respondents reported thinking that CBD is a type of 'miracle cure', over one-third stated that they weren't quite sure just what CBD is. The remaining respondents felt that CBD was just 'hype'. Furthermore, one-fourth of users said that they purchased CBD on impulse, 7% purchased CBD due to their physician's recommendation, and the remaining 60% stated that their first CBD purchase was planned.

These survey findings from early 2019 outline that there remains quite a gender gap between daily CBD users, and also indicates that there is a significant portion of users who are not quite sure what CBD is yet use it regardless. Hopefully, ongoing research will help dispel any confusion specific to CBD's use as well as its known effects.

Safety and side effects of CBD

CBD has been reported as being remarkably tolerable in humans[17], even at relatively high doses (e.g. 1500mg/day)[18]. And unlike many drugs, there does not appear to be a generated tolerance to CBD, indicating that those who use CBD for extended periods of time should not expect to have to increase their dose over time[19]. Still, when talking about safety or side effects of a consumable like CBD, we have to look a little deeper at what these terms represent. Defining 'tolerable' or 'safe' can be quite relative in nature depending on the individual. Some might consider 'safe' to mean no significant side effects such as drowsiness or a skin rash. To a person dying of a potentially terminal disease, however, 'safe' may be inferred as meaning that it won't cause their condition to worsen even though it might cause other negative effects such as skin rash or weight gain. Therefore, when looking at safety as well as potential side effects for a product such as CBD designed to improve health, it is important to establish a degree of context regarding what 'safe' represents relative to the medical condition that CBD is being taken for.

In looking for a benchmark that outlines a standard of safety for CBD, it's probably worthwhile to look at one of the more universal standards such as what has been outlined by the World Health Organization (WHO). In 2017 the WHO evaluated CBD and released a statement specific to the abuse potential of CBD in which it concluded that "[i]n humans, CBD exhibits no effects indicative of any abuse or dependence potential". Furthermore, the WHO evaluated the safety aspect of CBD and concluded that " . . . there is no evidence of recreational use of CBD or any public health-related problems associated with the use of pure CBD"[20].

Such findings should be considered to relay a degree of confidence specific to the relative safety of CBD. Truth be told, under the right circumstances almost any substance could be considered to have serious safety issues. Take peanuts for example – the vast majority of people can consume peanuts and associated products without concern. Still, a small portion of the population can have life-threatening events occur if they come into contact with a peanut – or even eat foods that were produced in a factory that also processed peanuts. As of yet, no known reports of CBD 'allergy' or severe reactions similar to what could happen with peanuts have been reported. There have, however, been reports of severe incidents from patients taking tainted synthetic cannabidiol[21], which should raise concern specific to the safety of this type of cannabidiol.

Side effects of CBD

Side effects relate to any unintended or unwanted events associated with taking a product such as CBD. Side effects of CBD use reported in healthy humans are typically anecdotal (i.e. based on personal experience rather than scientific study) in nature but are generally mild, reported as ranging from general malaise (feeling 'off') to drowsiness and/or fatigue[22]. In some cases, side effects can be related to the condition that the patient may have. For example, one study reported an increase in CBD-associated sedation among patients with schizophrenia given an oral dose[23]. However, sedation is not an expected finding in healthy patients taking CBD. Therefore, 'sedation' as a reported side effect of CBD may not be an expected occurrence – even in healthy individuals – as it has only been established scientifically in schizophrenic patients.

In animals, CBD has been shown to inhibit liver-based drug metabolism, diminish fertilization capability, and diminish certain drug transport protein functions (e.g. p-glycoproteins)[24]. Other reports, however, have shown that rodents taking CBD for two weeks in doses ranging from 3-30mg per kilogram (kg) of body weight did not show any clinical issues related to heart rate, blood pressure, glucose levels, sodium or potassium levels, or body temperature, nor did CBD use affect the movement of digested food through the intestine or alter psychological function[19]. What's more, CBD did not affect measures such as urine osmolality, pH, albumin, leukocyte, or erythrocyte counts[3]. And in mice taking a higher 60mg/kg CBD dose, postural effects such as kyphosis, a swaying gate, and tail stiffness were unchanged, as was muscle coordination (i.e. 'ataxia'), vocalization, and defecation[25].

80

Whether these effects could be considered as 'side effects' or 'effects' is up for debate, but again it is important to note that many of these events occurred in rodents. Rodents typically receive CBD through an oral dose or intraperitoneal (i.e. abdominal) injection. Humans, on the other hand, are generally studied using CBD administered via inhalation or through the oral pathway[10]. The differences in how a substance is administered may seem somewhat irrelevant, but it is in fact very important. For example, if a factor such as stomach acidity alters the molecular structure of an oral dose of CBD, that dose would in turn have no effect if the CBD was destroyed by the stomach acid. Therefore, it's imperative that research is able to outline the delivery and effectiveness of various administration routes of CBD to evaluate how much of a dose is actually delivered to the bloodstream. In other words, if someone is taking CBD for tinnitus, is there evidence that the dose of CBD using that specific dosing application (e.g. eardrops, oral) is making it to the bloodstream intact so that it can reach the tissue of interest and exert its effects on the tinnitus? Unfortunately, with many vestibular disorders such as Ménière's disease, vestibular migraine, or even tinnitus, there is a whole other argument to be made regarding CBD use as we don't yet know which tissues are involved in many of these conditions and thereby don't know which tissue to target for therapy.

When it comes to side effects of CBD, it is important to look for a potentially compounding aspect that may contribute to any noted side effects. THC is found (in very small doses) in some CBD products which brings up the question of whether a small THC amount may actually be the cause of – or at least contribute to – some of the reported side effects of CBD. One study from Germany set out to determine whether noted side effects of CBD could be due to interference from THC, with surprising results[22]. Of 28 CBD samples evaluated in the study, THC levels found in the analyzed samples warranted that –

according to European regulations – 36% of the tested samples be deemed as harmful to health and 50% of the samples should be considered as unfit for human consumption! Furthermore, the authors verified that any detected THC was not due to unintended conversion of CBD to THC, which can happen under certain circumstances[26]. As a result of these findings, the study's authors concluded that there was viable evidence to suggest that some reported side effects of CBD use may actually be due to THC ingestion.

Potential Drug Interactions

Alongside the topic of safety, it is also of interest to establish whether there is any type of interaction between CBD and pharmaceutical drugs which may be taken at the same time. Unfortunately, determining such effects requires extensive research to establish conclusively and may take years for each drug tested. Still, one author provided a degree of optimism in pointing out that other ingredients found in CBD oils are typically at such a low concentration that they should not be expected to cause a major interaction with other drugs[27]. Much work remains to be done in order to rule out potential drug interactions, but current evidence regarding CBD's safety in this area appears promising.

Specific to the mechanism of how CBD is metabolized by the body, like many pharmaceutical drugs CBD interacts with enzymes such as those in the cytochrome P450 group. Therefore, drugs that inhibit the activity of this enzyme group – such as ritonavir and clarithromycin – may also influence the metabolism of CBD given that CBD is metabolized by the CYP3A4 enzyme[28] which is itself a member of the P450 enzyme family. It is important to note, though, that this is a relatively common effect given that approximately 60% of pharmaceutical drugs are metabolized by the CYP3A4 enzyme[29]. Whereas CBD is also metabolized by this same enzyme, the potential – emphasis on *potential,* not on *risk* or *proof* – exists that some drug interaction may occur when taking CBD. Interestingly, this metabolic pathway invites the same set of problems that comes with consuming furanocoumarins – compounds found in grapefruit juice! Therefore, CBD may end up being associated with drugs assigned the so-called "grapefruit warning" which indicates that the drug should not be consumed with grapefruit juice. Such inhibition from grapefruit juice could mean a slower breakdown of CBD, in turn resulting in a higher overall dose of drugs taken concurrent with CBD[10]. Conversely, drugs such as phenobarbital or rifampicin increase the activity of CYP34A[28]. This increased activity has the potential to decrease the availability of CBD within the body due to an increased metabolism which effectively 'burns through' circulating CBD at a faster rate.

From another angle, CBD is known to inhibit the CYP2C19 enzyme[30]. Drugs such as hexobarbital that are metabolized by CYP2C19 may result in a higher level of hexobarbital in the body when the drug is taken with CBD[31]. Interestingly, this effect may have beneficial uses as well. In one study, CBD's interaction with CYP3A4 and CYP2C19 actually increased the bioavailability (i.e. active drug amount within the body) of clonazepam among children being treated for epilepsy[32]. While this may seem somewhat problematic at first, the interaction actually allowed for a reduced dosage to be administered, in turn reducing the side effects of clonazepam.

While we're on the topic of CBD's interaction with enzymes, it's worth mentioning that CBD has been shown to increase activity of the CYP1A1 enzyme. This particular enzyme is involved with the breakdown of materials that have been known to increase one's risk for developing cancer such as benzopyrene[10]. Therefore, it is hypothesized that CBD may indirectly play a role in helping the body avoid the absorption of certain problematic substances into the bloodstream[10].

CBD and THC

CBD's potential interaction with THC is of interest as it has been reported to help attenuate the psychological effects of THC[33]. This finding may help explain a past preference for cannabis plants which had the highest THC:CBD ratio[34] in order to ensure minimal CBD-based interference with any THC-related response. However, the recent explosion in CBD interest along with changing federal regulations specific to CBD allowances has now created a shift toward a more CBD-prominent product[35]. As discussed earlier, CBD is capable of being converted chemically to THC, but the process for doing so (acid-catalyzed cyclization) is more involved than other THC-synthesizing processes[26].

There appears to be an inverse relationship between the amount of THC and CBD present in cannabis plants[26]. Hemp flowers contain approximately 2% CBD; however, cannabis bred for recreational use contains 20% or more THC within its flowers[36]. In other parts of the world such as Switzerland, cannabis plant THC levels are permitted to reach 1%[34], much higher than the 0.3-0.7% considered as illegal by U.S. standards[36]. Interestingly, a THC level of approximately 1% is considered to be the point at which there is a potential for intoxication[26]; therefore, the 0.3% threshold required of hemp plants should prevent any expected psychogenic effects. Recently, pharmaceutical companies have been known to breed hemp capable of producing 20% CBD[36]. For medical purposes, the drug Sativex is produced using a specific THC:CBD ratio of 1:1[37], but this ratio was determined under scientific study to have the most beneficial results for the intended use of the drug.

Still, it must be recognized that all CBD plants produce some degree of THC at a ratio of 25:1 CBD:THC[36]. Because of difficulty in removing *all* THC from a strain, it further heightens the need for patients to be aware of potential THC contamination in samples that do not undergo chemical analysis. Too high of THC intake for too long can cause medical issues such as cannabinoid hyperemesis, but a quality CBD product in conjunction with chemical analysis should alleviate any THC-related concern.

Effects of CBD

Now that we've outlined several of the potential safety issues and side effects associated with CBD use, let's take a look at what the research has outlined specific to CBD's effects in the body. In this section we'll focus our attention on what has been shown to occur through research studies rather than discuss the many anecdotal effects of CBD that are often reported. This is certainly not to say that individual patient reports are not accurate; rather, we are going to stick with research results simply because the reported effects are shown to be specifically tied to CBD. In a later chapter we'll discuss the experimental process which helps outline the detail needed to report the effects of something like CBD. Then, you as a patient will be able to determine on your own whether the individual claims you hear at times about CBD are legitimate enough for you to pursue on your own.

Despite CBD initially being relegated to the proverbial 'back burner' in favor of THC, research from as far back as the 1970s revealed positive benefits from CBD. One of the earliest findings revealed how CBD can influence the THC response[38]. Unlike THC, CBD does not provide any psychotropic effects despite the fact that both CBD and THC are cannabinoids. This psychoactive quality of THC is largely due to differences within the molecular structure, as THC is capable of binding to the CB1 receptor while the primary form of CBD does not bind to CB1 and therefore does not have the same influence on the brain as THC[12]. Other early reports of CBD included an ability for CBD to positively influence certain cells in Nieman-Pick disease[39], a condition that influences fat metabolism and deposition. Studies from CBD's early days also revealed much about the anti-epileptic[40] and anti-anxiety features of CBD[41].

As CBD became more well-known, research started to reveal certain characteristics across studies that outlined the effects of CBD as both physiological and psychological in nature. The physiological responses reported in the research are quite substantial, though are largely limited to animal-based research. For example, four weeks of CBD use in obese mice was found to increase high-density lipoproteins (i.e. 'good' cholesterol) and decrease total cholesterol[42]. CBD was also shown to inhibit weight gain in rats as well as reduce drug-induced excessive eating behavior[43]. In mice prone to diabetes, CBD administration appeared to suppress the advancement of diabetes[44]. CBD's benefit as a potential anti-inflammatory was shown in results which indicated that four days of transdermal application of CBD in arthritic rats reduced joint swelling and other indicators of arthritis[45]. CBD has also been shown to work against methicillin-resistant *staphylococcus aureus* (MRSA)[46] and helps to reduce the risk of stroke[47]. Even certain anti-cancer effects have been revealed with CBD administration, including an inhibition of metastatic nodules[48], reduction of tumor metastasis[49], and a decrease in the number of polyps in colon-cancer-induced mice[50]. Of particular interest is that these treatments appeared to work without the unfortunate side effects that are associated with many cancer treatments.

Studying the psychological effects of CBD can invite a unique set of issues for researchers as psychological effects are largely reliant upon the measurement of patient-reported symptoms. Unlike 'signs', symptoms such as dizziness, nausea, or certain aspects of anxiety are difficult to be measured by an observer and therefore must be reported by the patient. For example – 'How dizzy are you today?' cannot be determined solely by a researcher, yet a patient can report their own dizziness rating by using a numeric value, such as 1-10. Trends can then be assessed over time to see if the reported dizziness value (e.g. "4") has changed in response to a particular treatment to see if there is an improvement. Animal research into psychological disorders, however, can be a bit more problematic. Rats or mice cannot rate their own depression or anxiety, so how can these symptoms be measured in the research? It is possible to be done using specially designed research models, but doing so creates *limitations to the model* that invites a bit of uncertainty in trying to ensure that the dizziness, anxiety, or other symptom was truly present.

In vestibular research, tinnitus is a symptom that cannot be measured by an observer; therefore, the degree and type of tinnitus is dependent upon the patient matching their tinnitus to a recording. To test a drug's effect on tinnitus in animals, it's not easy to determine a rat or mouse's level of tinnitus. Therefore, researchers looking at a particular drug (or CBD) have to find evidence that tinnitus appears to be occurring. One study developed a model for tinnitus-based research by training rodents to associate pure silence with a food reward[51]. Then they had some of those mice subjected to intense, loud noise for a period of time. Later, some mice did not seek the reward once the loud noise was eliminated, and it was inferred that those mice still experienced a perceived sound, which would be equivalent to tinnitus. But, a limitation of that model is that it was not known whether the mice truly had tinnitus, and so any effect of the studied drug treatment's ability to treat tinnitus could only be based on the inference that tinnitus was occurring.

Limitations are at times our only option, so when it comes to CBD and psychological effects, studies that show a reported effect in animals should not be excluded. For example, CBD has been shown to improve the emotional test response in depressed rats[52]. In chronically-stressed rats, CBD use was reported to reduce anxiety through a mechanism thought to be related to serotonin levels[53]. Another study found that high (60mg/kg) doses of CBD had similar effects to clonazepam[54], a drug used for several psychological conditions, and the CBD use did not appear to elicit any side effects. These purported psychological effects could be particularly beneficial for vestibular conditions such as persistent postural-perceptual dizziness (PPPD) which are thought to have considerable psychological input and are also known to be associated with anxiety[55].

Misconceptions of CBD Effects

While it is clear that CBD does have a significant effect on the body, there are also a lot of misconceptions about just what CBD is capable of doing. Therefore, let's take a moment to outline some of the more common misunderstandings surrounding CBD. For one, we have talked quite a bit about how THC is often labeled as a 'psychotropic' drug while CBD is typically considered the opposite – a 'non-psychotropic' drug. Though THC is certainly capable of producing psychogenic activity, one author pointed out that CBD's influence on mood disorders such as schizophrenia or even depression warrant discussion of CBD more as a 'non-intoxicating' drug than a non-psychotropic drug[4]. Along these same lines, CBD has been incorrectly labeled as having a sedative effect when in fact quite the opposite occurs, including CBD's ability to counteract the sedation that typically occurs with THC use[4]. It's only when

CBD is combined with small doses of THC for the treatment of epilepsy disorder that a sedative-type response is noted[56].

It is also a common misconception that CBD is undergoing extensive research testing in humans regarding its potential health benefits and therapeutic effects. Unfortunately, this isn't quite true. The only case in which CBD has undergone clinical trials in humans was for study of the drug Epidiolex® which was approved by the FDA for treatment of a rare form of epilepsy[27]. Using CBD in human research studies is quite complicated regarding federal regulations due to approval processes and approved providers. As such, there is not a directed interest at present to conduct CBD-related experiments on humans.

Another point to clarify specific to a common misconception about CBD is that *CBD is safe.* Under the right conditions, CBD has been shown to be a very safe product to use with minimal side effects. However, the explosion in CBD production and sales, combined with a relatively simple process for extracting CBD from the *cannabis sativa* plant, allows for what can often be an unchecked production process. Consequently, variations in CBD content as well as the possible inclusion of contaminants such as herbicides or even THC are possible in some less-reputable CBD products. Therefore, patients must be aware of the potential effects that any included contaminants may have on their health and look for CBD products that have undergone quality control checks.

A final point to make regarding a potential misconception is that CBD is legal, which is in fact true in most states as long as specific processing protocols are followed. However, depending upon the processing of CBD and any associated contaminants, there is a low but plausible risk of testing positive for THC on a drug test[57]. This risk is more related to the extraction process and subsequent contaminants, and should not be a concern with CBD obtained from manufacturers that provide analyses of their batch CBD runs. Still, some CBD suppliers note in disclaimers on their website that there is a risk when taking their product that a positive drug test may occur for THC. One company's qualifying statement for such a claim outlines that CBD and THC are difficult to distinguish on drug tests, and using CBD may result in a subsequent false-positive test. So, even though you may be taking a THC-free product, CBD suppliers warn of a risk of testing positive for THC due to some drug tests not being able to discriminate between THC and CBD.

Labeling Accuracy

When you buy any product, there is generally an expectation of honesty from you that the seller has assembled their product as advertised. With many manufactured products such as sporting equipment or electronics it is relatively easy to establish whether you 'got what you paid for' by simply using the product. Medications and supplements, however, aren't quite as clear cut given the fact that there's no way for the average consumer to establish whether each dose does indeed contain the proper amount of supplement, cannabinoid, etc. With drugs, the FDA handles the process of ensuring that manufacturers are selling the product as advertised, which is to say that each pill contains the amount of medication listed – within very tight constraints. CBD, however, is not manufactured or sold under the same rules as drugs. For example, CBD does not require a prescription for use like many pharmaceutical drugs do. Still, the FDA has also established that CBD does not fall under the umbrella of dietary supplements, either[58]. As we discussed earlier, the FDA has approved Epidiolex® – a drug which contains purified CBD – for seizures associated with certain diseases, but there are no other FDA-approved drug products that have CBD in the ingredient list[58].

Even though it contains the non-psychotropic component of cannabis, there is still quite a bit of regulation of CBD. In fact, it can get quite confusing for any individual to try and decipher. For example, you cannot at present legally sell a food to which CBD has been added[58]. Similarly, the FDA has made it clear that CBD cannot be marketed as a treatment or preventative for disease. In fact, several 'cease and desist' letters have been sent from the FDA to CBD producers requiring them to stop using such claims in their marketing. However, no one is known to have yet been subjected to enforcement action by the FDA regarding these claims.

The accuracy of the CBD label is imperative for patients. If the label overstates the quantity of CBD, for example, there is likely a diminished medical effect, if any medical effect exists at all. Conversely, if the label incorrectly understates the true CBD quantity in the container, there is not likely a medical risk to the patient given the relative safety of CBD[19, 59], but it does call into question the manufacturer's production practices such as whether it is performing quantitative analysis of their product prior to it being packaged for sale. Even with analysis, though, there can be discrepancies. Generally, the equipment used for analysis of CBD samples is dependent upon the lab performing the analysis. One study from 2011 found evidence that the type of equipment used for the analysis can result in variations in the reported CBD content. Gas chromatography analysis reported 20-33% higher CBD content than identical samples analyzed using high-pressure liquid chromatography[60], even though gas chromatography converts acidic cannabinoids to a neutral form as a result of the heat generated during analysis[34].

The variation that can occur with CBD product labeling was revealed by one study which evaluated 84 different online CBD products for labeling accuracy[59]. Analysis revealed that actual CBD product concentrations ranged from 0.10mg/ml to 655mg/ml. Of the analyzed products, only 30% were appropriately labeled, with 'appropriate' being considered as having an analyzed CBD content within 10% of the stated label quantity. Nearly half (43%) of the products contained at least 10% more CBD than stated on the label, while over one-fourth contained at least 10% less CBD than what was outlined on the label. Interestingly, oil-based CBD was the most consistently labeled, with 45% of oil-based CBD stating the accurate amount. Vape-style CBD was improperly labeled 88% of the time. Of note is that THC was detected at levels up to 6.43mg/ml in over 20% of the samples tested, which could be particularly problematic given the potential for noticeable effects in children[61].

Labeling accuracy has the potential to invite safety issues, but may also run afoul of federal regulations surrounding CBD. The FDA does take action at times when it finds that CBD label-based information does not match what is found in the product or does not fall within the proper guidelines. In 2019 the FDA sent out over 20 'warning letters' to manufacturers regarding aspects such as 'Dietary Supplement Labeling', 'Unapproved New Drugs', and 'Misbranded Drugs'[62]. For example, one letter addresses a company's 'dietary supplement labeling' of CBD such that:

" . . . you intend to market your (products) that contain CBD as dietary supplements. Specifically, your (products) bear the statement "Dietary Supplement" on their product labels. However, your products cannot be dietary supplements because they do not meet the definition of dietary supplement under section 201(ff) of the FD&C Act, 21 U.S.C. 321(ff). FDA has concluded, based on available evidence, that CBD products are excluded from the dietary supplement definition under sections 201(ff)(3)(B)(i) and (ii) of the FD&C Act, 21 U.S.C. 321(ff)(3)(B)(i) and (ii).

Similarly, under the 'Unapproved New Drug" policy, the FDA has warned:

> *Based on our review of your website, your (products) are drugs under section 201(g)(1) of the FD&C Act, 21 U.S.C. 321(g)(1), because they are intended for use in the diagnosis, cure, mitigation, treatment, or prevention of disease, and/or intended to affect the structure or any function of the body.*
>
> *Examples of claims observed on your website that establish the intended use of your products as drugs include, but may not be limited to, the following:*

On a webpage:

> - *"The fact that (product) CBD oil is THC-free & non-psychoactive makes it an appealing option for patients looking for relief from inflammation, pain, anxiety, psychosis, seizures, neurodegenerative diseases, spasm . . ."*

Your (products) are not generally recognized as safe and effective for the above referenced uses and, therefore, these products are "new drug[s]" under section 201(p) of the FD&C Act, 21 U.S.C. 321(p). New drugs may not be legally introduced or delivered for introduction into interstate commerce without prior approval from the FDA, as described in sections 301(d) and 505(a) of the FD&C Act, 21 U.S.C. 331(d) and 355(a). FDA approves a new drug on the basis of scientific data and information demonstrating that the drug is safe and effective. There are no FDA-approved applications in effect for your products.

Perhaps as an indicator of the growth of CBD-related products in just the past couple of years, 22 total FDA warning letters were sent out in 2019, a stark increase over a single letter being sent out in 2018 and only four letters sent in 2017[62]. Therein lies the main argument when it comes to CBD regulation: it is confusing! It may be due to the relatively new status of CBD in the medical playing field, or the fact that CBD has medical and non-medical uses, or it may simply be due to

93

the fact that government regulations seem destined to remain confusing. On the one hand, CBD has been shown to reduce or prevent the occurrence of seizures in some childhood conditions that do not respond to anti-seizure medication[63]. Therefore, CBD seems to have the effects of a medication, and given the severe effects of seizures, CBD in some cases may indeed best be handled under the supervision of a physician.

In what may be an attempt to guard against increasingly risky situations like those related to seizures, the DEA has assigned a code for 'marihuana extract' to the list of Schedule-1 (i.e. no medical benefit, high potential for abuse) drugs as follows:

> "Meaning an extract containing one or more cannabinoids that has been derived from any plant of the genus Cannabis, other than the separated resin (whether crude or purified) obtained from the plant."

As written, this statement does not clearly list CBD but does make it clear that an extract containing cannabinoids is listed in Schedule-1 of the Code of Federal Regulations. To be clear, all cannabinoids are considered as *derivatives* or *components* of marijuana[64].

In your search through CBD products you will no doubt come across terms on labels or in marketing tools which tout claims such as "high-CBD" or "low-THC strain". Be aware, however, that there is no universally-accepted definition for what these terms mean[64]. In other words, selling a 'high-CBD' oil doesn't mean that there is a particular content, concentration, or ratio of CBD in the product. These phrases can easily be used as sales pitches without providing clear evidence, so as a savvy consumer and patient you must ensure that what you are buying is actually comprised of what the seller claims.

The CBD extraction process

Within the cannabis plant, cannabinoids themselves are located primarily in the flower of the plant and, to a lesser degree, the leaves[65]. To get CBD from these parts of the plant into a form that can be utilized by the endocannabinoid system, it must be removed, or *extracted*, from the plant using a process capable of separating the cannabinoid from the other portions of the plant and then getting the extracted CBD into a useable form. The process of removing the cannabinoids can be summed up as a set of steps that involves crushing the dried plant material, exposing it to a liquid, and then removing the excess or unnecessary materials (e.g. plant remnants). Once the extract has been removed and concentrated, it is then mixed with an edible oil (e.g. olive, vegetable, etc.) to produce the final marketed product. The one exception to this is the oil-extraction process, which utilizes an oil product such as olive or vegetable oil to perform the extraction process itself, after which it is filtered and ready for sale.

The function of each extraction technique is largely dependent upon the solubility of CBD or other cannabinoid within the extraction solvent of choice which can include methanol, ethanol, butane, or hexane, among others[66]. It is important to point out that this process removes *all* biologically active compounds from the plant including other phytocannabinoids, terpenes, and omega-3 fatty acids[67]. Such extracts are often marketed as 'full-spectrum' due to containing 'all' beneficial extract components[27]. Subsequent processing can isolate individual components of the plant if the manufacturer chooses.

While the amount of CBD capable of being produced from each process has been outlined using very specific techniques, methods such as ethanol extraction do invite the opportunity for user error. For example, using too high of heat during an ethanol evaporation is reported to have the potential to denature the CBD[68]. Such complications are particularly important for consumers given that these complications can affect the CBD content of the extract; therefore it is again recommended that CBD be bought only from reputable suppliers that provide a chemical analysis (e.g. mass spectrophotometry) of *each lot* – not just of their original production run.

Think about the importance of chemical analysis this way – if you buy the cheapest CBD oil available, and that supply happens to be produced by an individual in his or her basement using a mortar and pestle in conjunction with an oil extraction, what guarantee do you have as to the quantity of CBD per dose in that particular bottle? Pharmaceutical drug manufacturers

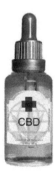

Figure 3.1. Here is a relatively nondescript bottle of CBD oil. There is no way to visually confirm the presence of CBD in this bottle - only a chemical analysis will provide that vital information

are required to prove consistent dosing prior to selling their product; however, CBD (and supplement manufacturers) are not. Without specific testing of the product in order to quantify the true dose in a bulk preparation, there is no way as a consumer or patient to ensure that you are even getting *any* CBD in your product. Factors such as the aforementioned user error, measurement inconsistencies, or dilution amounts can all affect the final dosing. Without evidence and/or certification of what you are purchasing, combined with the fact that many patients do not feel the actual effects of their CBD during treatment, there is no way to ensure that what you paid for is actually what you received. Therefore, you as the patient should be able to confirm with the CBD producer the actual quantity – usually in mg/ml (milligrams per milliliter) – of the very product run from which you bought. This will likely result in a higher-priced product due to the costs associated with additional testing, but at the same time you are ensuring quality specific to the CBD content of what you purchased.

Specific to extraction procedures, several methods can be used, each with a degree of positive or negative benefits and potentially even risks (e.g. explosion). For example, one procedure involves ultrasonic extraction and can be used with minimal application of heat, a particular benefit given that heat has the potential to damage cannabinoid structures[69]. One of the more validated extraction methods involves the use of carbon dioxide (CO_2), a technique which is commonly used in the production of extracts such as essential oils[70] as well as in extracting oil from hemp seeds[66]. Hemp itself is low in cannabinoid content at approximately 4% or less[34] which in turn led to development of CO_2 extraction from the cannabis plant that has been reported to be both cheaper and more ecological[71]. Next, we'll look at the most common extraction techniques in order to outline how CBD is removed from the plant and processed into its commonly marketed forms.

CO₂ extraction

To complete the CO_2 extraction process, plant leaves and buds are ground up and subjected to supercritical, pressurized CO2 for several hours. 'Supercritical' indicates that the CO_2 is at a precise point where it exists as both a gas and liquid state. This in turn allows the gas portion of the CO_2 to diffuse through the plant particles to aid in cannabinoid extraction while the liquid portion carries the extracted material out. Upon depressurization of the CO_2, cannabinoids and other materials within the mixture precipitate out from the remaining material, after which the CO_2 is removed so as to leave the extract behind.

After processing with CO_2, exposing the resulting resin to a sub-zero-degree solvent allows additional materials (e.g. fatty or waxy resins) to be removed, further refining and purifying the extract in a process commonly called 'winterization'. If desired, further refinement of the extract can be performed to allow for separation of specific cannabinoids. Chemical analysis such as high-performance liquid chromatography (HPLC) can then be used to establish the actual cannabinoid content of the extract[66].

While very effective at extracting cannabinoids from the plant, the use of supercritical CO_2 as an extraction method involves a significant investment of equipment (estimated at $40,000[68]) as well as expertise in use of that equipment. However, the CO_2 extraction process is reported to produce a high cannabinoid yield with good efficiency[66].

Solvent Extraction

Solvent extraction of cannabinoids involves a relatively simple process and much less expensive equipment than CO_2 extraction. With solvent extraction, ground-up plant particles are mixed with ethanol, after which the ethanol is strained to remove the plant mass. The remaining liquid is then slowly heated which serves to evaporate off the ethanol, leaving only the extract that contains all solubilized plant materials such as cannabinoids and terpenes.

Ice Water Extraction

Ice water extraction is another relatively simple process and also presents less injury risk potential than the solvent extraction procedures that utilize volatile chemicals. With ice water extraction, ground up plant components are combined with ice (or dry ice), after which water is added and the material is mixed for a period of time. The plant mass is then strained from the mixture while the extract, which contains all of the solubilized material, is allowed to separate from the water prior to being mixed with an oil to create the final product.

Oil Extraction

Oil extraction produces a final, quite diluted 'oil' rather than a true 'extract', but is rather simple to perform. Of note, however, is that the true concentration of CBD within this preparation is dependent upon the amount of oil used in the process as well as the effectiveness of the extraction. To perform oil extraction, ground-up plant particles are suspended in an edible oil (e.g. olive, vegetable) and warmed for a 1-2 hour period. The mixture is then strained, leaving an extract-rich oil that can immediately be packaged for use.

CBD Delivery methods

At this point we have covered two of the three primary components of what is involved in understanding CBD. First of all, we outlined the cannabidiol itself, which is found primarily in the cannabis flowers and to a lesser degree in the leaves. The second component was to describe the extraction process, which results in CBD being dissolved in some type of solvent (e.g. ethanol) or supercritical fluid like prepared CO_2. The third step, which we'll cover next, is to outline the process for getting the CBD into a format (e.g. topical, edible) that can deliver the CBD into the body so that it can exert its benefits.

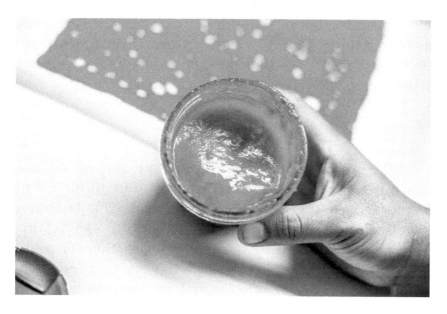

Figure 4.2. The CBD extraction process produces a thick, waxy substance that must then be diluted with oil or other substance in order to get the CBD into a deliverable form

The use of an edible oil to dissolve the extract is one of the most common methods for CBD delivery. Benefits of using oil include its ability to be used in a consumable form, its relatively simply dosing method such as in using a 'teaspoon' or in counting total 'drops' applied, and the absence of odor that might identify an individual as a CBD user as may occur with smoking or vaporizing (i.e. "vaping") CBD[72]. Furthermore, the use of oil is relatively economical given that once the extract is dissolved in oil, CBD is typically in a marketable format that is commonly found on store shelves. However, much like solvent preferences, the oil used can differ across CBD producers. Sunflower, hemp, olive[72], and even coconut oil[64] are commonly utilized to dissolve the extract into a useable delivery method.

Besides oil, other CBD-based products include pills, balms, e-cigarettes, and 'edibles' that consist of products such as gummy bears. However, it is important to remember that the use of CBD in food or supplement products is strictly prohibited in the United States by the FDA (though allowed in Canada). Current allowances toward CBD being sold in edibles is more due to a lack of federal enforcement than due to it being legal[73].

Topical application

The topical application of CBD products is typically found in items such as balms developed from materials like beeswax. It is known that cannabinoids can be absorbed through the skin[26]; therefore the potential for topical application as a means to get cannabinoids into the body is viable. However, it is also important to examine whether the carrier material (e.g. patch gel, lotion, oil, etc.) that holds the suspended or solubilized CBD is capable of being absorbed through the skin. If the carrier used cannot cross through the skin, the CBD cannot effectively reach the bloodstream.

Drops or sprays

Oil-based tinctures are manufactured as a means to deliver CBD directly into the mouth. This method of delivery is often recommended to be held under the tongue for 30-90 seconds to allow for direct entry into the bloodstream. Swallowing the oil is also acceptable, though doing so will delay entry of the CBD into the bloodstream due to it having to first pass through the digestive system.

Edibles (including pills)

Certain manufacturers provide food products infused with CBD. Unlike inhaled or topically applied CBD, consumed CBD will have to pass through the digestive system to enter the bloodstream; consequently, edible-based CBD will take longer to exert any effect(s). Furthermore, there is the possibility that the food product itself may affect the absorption of the CBD, and that certain activities such as exercise or illness may impact the absorption speed or amount from the intestines.

Inhalation

Inhalation such as vaporization (i.e. 'vaping') of CBD most commonly occurs by using a tool such as a vaping pen to vaporize CBD-infused liquid which is then inhaled. Typically, the liquid is contained within a unit termed a *cartridge* which contains the CBD combined with a thinning agent to produce a liquid. The cartridge is then inserted inside a battery-operated *vape pen* which raises the temperature of the liquid to the point that it turns into a vapor which can then be inhaled. One benefit of vaping is that it provides a rapid introduction of CBD into the bloodstream.

CBD dosing

Delivery of any medication or supplement occurs through what is known as a dose. For therapeutic medications, doses are determined by the manufacturer after a wealth of testing on living cells, animals, and eventually humans. Technical-sounding terms outlining characteristics of the medication are often discussed when a manufacturer establishes a dose, such as dose-response curve, half-life, onset of action, or LD_{50}. For CBD, the dosing recommendations for most CBD users are largely arbitrary in nature, based more often on trial-and-error than on actual scientific testing. This is understandable given that the scientific process is quite slow (as we'll discuss in a later chapter) and CBD has only gained steam within the market in the past few years. Therefore, data on factors such as dose-response just haven't had time to develop.

Such inexact CBD dosing recommendations are quite different from the federal requirements that must be met for a pharmaceutical drug to make it to market. Before being allowed to be sold, drugs must go through years of testing to establish side effects, drug interactions, dosing recommendations, expiration dates, and storage conditions. And, pharmaceutical drugs have to be tested on a wide range of people and on people with various other medical conditions in order to determine whether there is any concerning interaction with their primary drug. On one hand, maybe it's a good thing that CBD doesn't have to slug through this same approval process as a new drug – after all, the average drug takes 10-12 years to make it to the market, at an average expense of over $2 ½ billion[74]. The consequence of insufficient regulation for products like CBD, however, is a market that can run unchecked with imposters, false labeling, and safety risks.

When it comes to determining proper dosing recommendations for CBD, a major principle is focused on the issue of delivering enough active ingredient – in this case CBD – to survive the normal biological processes (such as digestion) to then make it into the bloodstream in a high enough amount for the CBD to exert favorable effects, all while avoiding significant side/adverse effects.   Looking back again at pharmaceutical drugs, final dosing amounts are determined through a long trial-and-error process that is first worked out on paper, then performed on individual cells, then on animals, then on humans to find a balance between what amount of drug is enough to effectively work on the problem (e.g. pain, insulin production, etc.) without causing unnecessary harm to the average patient.

Dosing recommendations are often determined by having a patient take a drug or substance such as CBD through one of the available delivery methods, followed by a blood analysis to determine how much of the active form of that drug can be found in the patient's bloodstream (known as *bioavailability*) and for how long. At present, however, this type of analysis has not been established for general CBD use. Rather, a variety of dosing recommendations are provided for CBD, but typically with the caveat that the ultimate dosing responsibility lies with you the patient. One report summarized some of the difficulties involved with setting a particular dosing schedule for CBD, with factors such as complexities involving cannabinoid pharmacology, any existing CBD:THC ratio, the degree of additional compounds found in cannabis, varying routes of administration, individual tolerance levels, and individual differences in cannabinoid metabolism as key factors[75].

Thankfully, CBD appears to be quite safe even at doses up to 1500mg/day[18]. Still, inconsistencies regarding dosing are rampant online.   Recommendations can be listed anywhere from less than 1mg up to 200mg four times daily. Even the relatively reliable website webmd.com currently provides only physician-supervised dosing recommendations for a particular medical condition which has been shown to respond favorably to CBD and has also gone under extensive scientific testing. For most CBD uses, however, listed recommendations aren't specific to any particular medical condition and also don't account for aspects such as patient weight (which would be listed as CBD amount *per kilogram of body weight*, typically) or whether other medication is being taken. Furthermore, most CBD sites don't provide a basis for their dosing recommendations such as would be shown via research studies or even patient testimonials. A few sites do mention starting at lower doses and then working up to the point where relief is found, but even the initial dose in those cases has a wide range, with anything from 1mg to 40mg or more recommended. Therefore, it must be said again that in most cases, CBD dosing recommendations are ultimately going to be left up to the discretion of the patient rather than a specific amount determined through scientific study as occurs with pharmaceutical drugs.

Another consistent commentary on most CBD websites is a point that 'not everyone responds the same to CBD'. While this is true, such a statement can also serve as a sort of disclaimer to help protect the seller by ensuring that they have leverage to state *"we never promised you it would work!"*. Interestingly, some CBD websites attribute the lack of a quick therapeutic response to a need to build up the CBD in your body, and it is often pointed out that you as a patient will need to use this initial time to experiment with different dosages to find what works for you. While true – and as we know there are many pharmaceutical drugs that often don't have a noticeable effect – the instructions to continue on with your CBD despite no noticeable effects highlights the importance of obtaining your CBD from a reputable supplier who is willing to verify the actual CBD content of your purchased stock. Otherwise, the lack of response that you might experience with a certain purchase may not be due to your improper dosing tactics but rather due to the fact that there is an inadequate amount of CBD even in your purchased product!

It is also important when dosing to ensure that your dose is specific to *you*. If the dose is not specifically laid out by the manufacturer or by your medical professional, don't start out at a dosing regimen that your friend uses, even if he or she is taking CBD for the same ailment. Similarly, don't assume that your dose is the same as your friend's if the CBD was manufactured at two separate facilities. Once again, unless each bottle's true analysis of CBD content can be accessed, there is no actual guarantee of CBD content; rather, the amount of CBD in a dose must merely be assumed.

One study did look at a dose-response relationship when taking 150mg, 300mg, 600mg, or placebo of CBD for anxiety, but the outcome measures were not chemical analysis of the participants' blood but rather clinical measures such as self-reported anxiety levels, blood pressure, and heart rate[76]. Interestingly, it was determined that 300mg of CBD reduced anxiety better than the other doses. Another group broke up oral dosing in children less than 100 pounds such that 'medically sensitive' patients should begin at 0.25mg/lb/day and 'medically non-sensitive' patients can use 0.5mg/lb/day divided across 2 to 3 doses per day[77]. However, scientific evidence for these dosing amounts was not listed; rather, the doses were reported to be derived from client data.

We touched on the following point when discussing the differences in testing humans versus animals, but it's worth mentioning again. The route of administration, which refers to how CBD is introduced into your body, is an important factor when it comes to dosing. For example, oral administration of CBD may require a higher dose due to the digestive process potentially compromising a good degree of the original dose.

Inhalation, which circumvents the digestive process and results in a quicker introduction of CBD into the bloodstream, may allow for lower dosing than oral administration, as might transdermal or sublingual application as well. It's tough to say specifically which method should be used for certain conditions because there is not an established CBD dosage for many medical conditions. Therefore, a patient may find that he or she needs a high topical dose that is different than what they would take with an oral dose.

The trial-and-error system is at play with dosing but is somewhat dependent upon the route of administration a patient chooses to use for their particular type of CBD. Think of it this way – if a bottle of CBD oil is labeled as '100mg of CBD' and has 20 milliliters (ml) of oil in the bottle, it is pertinent as a patient to know how much should be used per dose along with which route of administration should be used to obtain that dose. For example, using the above 20ml bottle, if a 1ml dose was recommended, it would supply 5mg of CBD. However, if a 20mg dose of CBD was recommended, it would require a 4ml application from that bottle. Therefore, it is best to spend time reviewing the CBD manufacturer recommendations for each product as well as discussing the appropriate dose with your medical professional.

An important point to make regarding dosing is that a product's available dose of CBD has been shown to be dependent upon storage conditions. For example, even in a relatively cold environment (e.g. 4°C), CBD concentration has been shown to decrease in an oil preparation during its initial six weeks[69]. Research has not yet established whether a longer storage further diminishes the concentration or whether temperature can halt or worsen this decrease. Still, evidence of a diminished CBD concentration even in relatively favorable storage conditions emphasizes the need for you as a consumer to be aware of when your particular batch of CBD was prepared so as to ensure that it is used prior to any potential for diminished CBD quantity.

Conclusion

Despite its relatively short history in the medical world, CBD has shown quite a bit of promise as a potential therapeutic agent. After decades spent in the shadows of THC, CBD has emerged to reveal several potential health-related characteristics including anti-inflammatory and anti-anxiety properties as well as many cellular responses. Within the cannabis plant, CBD is predominantly found in the flowers along with other components including terpenes and THC. Extraction of CBD and these other components can be performed using a variety of techniques, each of which employs specific procedures that capitalize on the particular extraction material. Given that there is a high potential for non-CBD components to be present within their purchased product, patients should seek out manufacturers who perform an analysis of each batch of CBD produced. Because of the variation in total CBD extraction that can occur, CBD dose is dependent upon several factors which include the concentration of the product and the route of administration that the particular CBD product requires. Ultimately, it is up to you the patient – through consultation with your medical professional – to determine the best CBD dose as well as the proper route of administration for your specific medical condition.

Chapter References

1. Adams, R., M. Hunt, and J. Clark, *Structure of cannabidiol, a product isolated from the marihuana extract of Minnesota wild hemp. I.* Journal of the American Chemical Society, 1940. **62**(1): p. 196-200.

2. Mechoulam, R. and Y. Shvo, *Hashish—I: the structure of cannabidiol.* Tetrahedron, 1963. **19**(12): p. 2073-2078.

3. Peres, F.F., V. Almeida, and V.C. Abilio, *Cannabidiol: An Overview of its Antipsychotic Properties*, in *Handbook of Cannabis and Related Pathologies.* 2017, Elsevier. p. 787-794.

4. Russo, E.B., *Cannabidiol claims and misconceptions.* Trends in pharmacological sciences, 2017. **38**(3): p. 198-201.

5. Ottersen, T., et al., *The crystal and molecular structure of cannabidiol.* Acta Chemica Scandinavica B, 1977. **31**: p. 807-812.

6. Thomas, A., et al., *Cannabidiol displays unexpectedly high potency as an antagonist of CB1 and CB2 receptor agonists in vitro.* British journal of pharmacology, 2007. **150**(5): p. 613-623.

7. Russo, E.B., *Taming THC: potential cannabis synergy and phytocannabinoid-terpenoid entourage effects.* British journal of pharmacology, 2011. **163**(7): p. 1344-1364.

8. Fogaça, M.V., A.C. Campos, and F.S. Guimarães, *Cannabidiol and 5-HT1A Receptors*, in *Neuropathology of Drug Addictions and Substance Misuse.* 2016, Elsevier. p. 749-759.

9. Guzman, F., *5-TH1A receptors in psychopharmacology.* Psychopharmacology Institute, 2019.

10. Iffland, K. and F. Grotenhermen, *An update on safety and side effects of cannabidiol: a review of clinical data and relevant animal studies.* Cannabis and cannabinoid research, 2017. **2**(1): p. 139-154.

11. White, H.L. and R.L. Tansik, *Effects of Δ9-tetrahydrocannabinol and cannabidiol on phospholipase and other enzymes regulating arachidonate metabolism.* Prostaglandins and Medicine, 1980. **4**(6): p. 409-417.

12. Burstein, S., *Cannabidiol (CBD) and its analogs: a review of their effects on inflammation.* Bioorganic & medicinal chemistry, 2015. **23**(7): p. 1377-1385.

13. Jagielski, D., *The Retail Market Will Make Up More Than 60% of CBD Sales in the U.S. by 2024*, in *The Motley Fool.* 2019.

14. Williams, S. *U.S. CBD Sales to Grow an Average of 107% Annually Through 2023*. 2019.

15. Brenan, M. *14% of Americans Say They Use CBD Products*. 2019.

16. Datatrek Research. *CBD Usage by Demographhics*. 2019.

17. Mechoulam, R., L.A. Parker, and R. Gallily, *Cannabidiol: an overview of some pharmacological aspects*. The Journal of Clinical Pharmacology, 2002. **42**(S1): p. 11S-19S.

18. Zuardi, A.W., et al., *Antipsychotic effect of cannabidiol*. The Journal of clinical psychiatry, 1995.

19. Machado Bergamaschi, M., et al., *Safety and side effects of cannabidiol, a Cannabis sativa constituent*. Current drug safety, 2011. **6**(4): p. 237-249.

20. Organization, W.H. *Cannabidiol (CBD) Pre-Review Report Agenda Item 5.2*. in *Expert Committee on Drug Dependence Thirty-ninth Meeting, Geneva*. 2017.

21. Kuehn, B., *Synthetic cannabidiol poisoning*. Jama, 2018. **319**(22): p. 2264-2264.

22. Lachenmeier, D.W., et al., *Are side effects of cannabidiol (CBD) products caused by tetrahydrocannabinol (THC) contamination?* F1000Research, 2019. **8**(1394): p. 1394.

23. Boggs, D.L., et al., *The effects of cannabidiol (CBD) on cognition and symptoms in outpatients with chronic schizophrenia a randomized placebo controlled trial*. Psychopharmacology, 2018. **235**(7): p. 1923-1932.

24. Holland, M., et al., *The effects of cannabinoids on P-glycoprotein transport and expression in multidrug resistant cells*. Biochemical pharmacology, 2006. **71**(8): p. 1146-1154.

25. Dirikoc, S., et al., *Nonpsychoactive cannabidiol prevents prion accumulation and protects neurons against prion toxicity*. Journal of Neuroscience, 2007. **27**(36): p. 9537-9544.

26. Small, E., *Evolution and classification of Cannabis sativa (marijuana, hemp) in relation to human utilization*. The botanical review, 2015. **81**(3): p. 189-294.

27. VanDolah, H.J., B.A. Bauer, and K.F. Mauck. *Clinicians' guide to cannabidiol and hemp oils*. in *Mayo Clinic Proceedings*. 2019. Elsevier.

28. Monographie, N., *Cannabidiol*. Deutscher Arzneimittel-Codex (DAC) inkl. Neues Rezeptur-Formularium (NRF). DAC/NRF October, 2015. **22**.

29. Guengerich, F.P., *Cytochrome P450 proteins and potential utilization in biodegradation.* Environmental health perspectives, 1995. **103**(suppl 5): p. 25-28.

30. Pelkonen, O., et al., *Inhibition and induction of human cytochrome P450 (CYP) enzymes.* Xenobiotica, 1998. **28**(12): p. 1203-1253.

31. Ujváry, I. and L. Hanuš, *Human metabolites of cannabidiol: a review on their formation, biological activity, and relevance in therapy.* Cannabis and Cannabinoid Research, 2016. **1**(1): p. 90-101.

32. Geffrey, A.L., et al., *Drug–drug interaction between clobazam and cannabidiol in children with refractory epilepsy.* Epilepsia, 2015. **56**(8): p. 1246-1251.

33. Pisanti, S., et al., *Cannabidiol: State of the art and new challenges for therapeutic applications.* Pharmacology & therapeutics, 2017. **175**: p. 133-150.

34. Hädener, M., S. König, and W. Weinmann, *Quantitative determination of CBD and THC and their acid precursors in confiscated cannabis samples by HPLC-DAD.* Forensic science international, 2019. **299**: p. 142-150.

35. ElSohly, M.A., et al., *Changes in cannabis potency over the last 2 decades (1995–2014): analysis of current data in the United States.* Biological psychiatry, 2016. **79**(7): p. 613-619.

36. Chandra, S., et al., *Cannabis cultivation: methodological issues for obtaining medical-grade product.* Epilepsy & Behavior, 2017. **70**: p. 302-312.

37. Marcu, J.P., *An overview of major and minor phytocannabinoids,* in *Neuropathology of drug addictions and substance misuse.* 2016, Elsevier. p. 672-678.

38. Karniol, I.G., et al., *Cannabidiol interferes with the effects of Δ9-tetrahydrocannabinol in man.* European journal of pharmacology, 1974. **28**(1): p. 172-177.

39. Burstein, S., S.A. Hunter, and L. Renzulli, *Stimulation of sphingomyelin hydrolysis by cannabidiol in fibroblasts from a Niemann-Pick patient.* Biochemical and biophysical research communications, 1984. **121**(1): p. 168-173.

40. Cunha, J.M., et al., *Chronic administration of cannabidiol to healthy volunteers and epileptic patients.* Pharmacology, 1980. **21**(3): p. 175-185.

41. Guimarães, F.S., et al., *Antianxiety effect of cannabidiol in the elevated plus-maze.* Psychopharmacology, 1990. **100**(4): p. 558-559.

42.   Jadoon, K.A., et al., *Efficacy and safety of cannabidiol and tetrahydrocannabivarin on glycemic and lipid parameters in patients with type 2 diabetes: a randomized, double-blind, placebo-controlled, parallel group pilot study.* Diabetes Care, 2016. **39**(10): p. 1777-1786.

43.   Scopinho, A.A., et al., *Cannabidiol inhibits the hyperphagia induced by cannabinoid-1 or serotonin-1A receptor agonists.* Pharmacology Biochemistry and Behavior, 2011. **98**(2): p. 268-272.

44.   Weiss, L., et al., *Cannabidiol arrests onset of autoimmune diabetes in NOD mice.* Neuropharmacology, 2008. **54**(1): p. 244-249.

45.   Hammell, D., et al., *Transdermal cannabidiol reduces inflammation and pain-related behaviours in a rat model of arthritis.* European Journal of Pain, 2016. **20**(6): p. 936-948.

46.   Appendino, G., et al., *Antibacterial cannabinoids from Cannabis sativa: a structure– activity study.* Journal of natural products, 2008. **71**(8): p. 1427-1430.

47.   Mishima, K., et al., *Cannabidiol prevents cerebral infarction via a serotonergic 5-hydroxytryptamine1A receptor–dependent mechanism.* Stroke, 2005. **36**(5): p. 1071-1076.

48.   Leanza, L., et al., *Pharmacological targeting of ion channels for cancer therapy: in vivo evidences.* Biochimica et Biophysica Acta (BBA)-Molecular Cell Research, 2016. **1863**(6): p. 1385-1397.

49.   Murase, R., et al., *Id-1 gene and protein as novel therapeutic targets for metastatic cancer.* 2012, AACR.

50.   Aviello, G., et al., *Chemopreventive effect of the non-psychotropic phytocannabinoid cannabidiol on experimental colon cancer.* Journal of molecular medicine, 2012. **90**(8): p. 925-934.

51.   Zheng, Y., P. Reid, and P.F. Smith, *Cannabinoid CB1 receptor agonists do not decrease, but may increase acoustic trauma-induced tinnitus in rats.* Frontiers in Neurology, 2015. **6**: p. 60.

52.   Linge, R., et al., *Cannabidiol induces rapid-acting antidepressant-like effects and enhances cortical 5-HT/glutamate neurotransmission: role of 5-HT1A receptors.* Neuropharmacology, 2016. **103**: p. 16-26.

53.   Schiavon, A.P., et al., *Influence of single and repeated cannabidiol administration on emotional behavior and markers of cell proliferation and neurogenesis in non-stressed mice.*

Progress in Neuro-Psychopharmacology and Biological Psychiatry, 2016. **64**: p. 27-34.

54. Gomes, F.V., et al., *Cannabidiol attenuates sensorimotor gating disruption and molecular changes induced by chronic antagonism of NMDA receptors in mice.* International Journal of Neuropsychopharmacology, 2015. **18**(5).

55. Popkirov, S., J.P. Staab, and J. Stone, *Persistent postural-perceptual dizziness (PPPD): a common, characteristic and treatable cause of chronic dizziness.* Practical neurology, 2018. **18**(1): p. 5-13.

56. Devinsky, O., et al., *Cannabidiol in patients with treatment-resistant epilepsy: an open-label interventional trial.* The Lancet Neurology, 2016. **15**(3): p. 270-278.

57. Greenwich Biosciences Inc, *Highlights of Prescribing Information*, E.c.o. solution, Editor. 2018.

58. Food, U. and D. Administration, *FDA regulation of cannabis and cannabis-derived products: questions and answers.* 2019.

59. Bonn-Miller, M.O., et al., *Labeling accuracy of cannabidiol extracts sold online.* Jama, 2017. **318**(17): p. 1708-1709.

60. Gieringer, D. and A. Hazekamp, *How accurate is potency testing.* O'Shaughnessy's, 2011. **17**.

61. Crippa, J.A., et al., *Δ9-THC intoxication by cannabidiol-enriched cannabis extract in two children with refractory epilepsy: full remission after switching to purified cannabidiol.* Frontiers in pharmacology, 2016. **7**: p. 359.

62. United States Food and Drug Administration. *Warning Letters and Test Results for Cannabidiol-Related Products.* 2019.

63. Zaheer, S., et al., *Epilepsy and Cannabis: A Literature Review.* Cureus, 2018. **10**(9).

64. Mead, A., *The legal status of cannabis (marijuana) and cannabidiol (CBD) under US law.* Epilepsy & Behavior, 2017. **70**: p. 288-291.

65. Hemp Industries Association. *Hemp Industries Association Publishes Statement in Response to Misbranding of Cannabidiol Products as 'Hemp Oil'.* 2014.

66. Rovetto, L.J. and N.V. Aieta, *Supercritical carbon dioxide extraction of cannabinoids from Cannabis sativa L.* The Journal of Supercritical Fluids, 2017. **129**: p. 16-27.

67. Citti, C., et al., *Medicinal cannabis: Principal cannabinoids concentration and their stability evaluated by a high performance liquid chromatography coupled to diode array and quadrupole time of flight mass spectrometry method.* Journal of

pharmaceutical and biomedical analysis, 2016. **128**: p. 201-209.
68.   PowerBlanket. *CBD Extraction Methods*. 2019.
69.   Calvi, L., et al., *Comprehensive quality evaluation of medical Cannabis sativa L. inflorescence and macerated oils based on HS-SPME coupled to GC–MS and LC-HRMS (q-exactive orbitrap®) approach.* Journal of pharmaceutical and biomedical analysis, 2018. **150**: p. 208-219.
70.   Reverchon, E. and I. De Marco, *Supercritical fluid extraction and fractionation of natural matter.* The Journal of Supercritical Fluids, 2006. **38**(2): p. 146-166.
71.   Perrotin-Brunel, H., et al., *Solubility of cannabinol in supercritical carbon dioxide.* Journal of Chemical & Engineering Data, 2010. **55**(9): p. 3704-3707.
72.   Hazekamp, A., *The trouble with CBD oil.* Medical cannabis and cannabinoids, 2018. **1**(1): p. 65-72.
73.   Lachenmeier, D., V. Bock, and A. Deych, *Hemp food products-an update.* Deut Lebensm Rundsch, 2019. **115**: p. 351-372.
74.   Avorn, J., *The \$2.6 billion pill—methodologic and policy considerations.* New England Journal of Medicine, 2015. **372**(20): p. 1877-1879.
75.   Abramovici, H., *Information for health care professionals: cannabis (marihuana, marijuana) and the cannabinoids.* Health Canada, 2013.
76.   Linares, I.M., et al., *Cannabidiol presents an inverted U-shaped dose-response curve in a simulated public speaking test.* Brazilian Journal of Psychiatry, 2019. **41**(1): p. 9-14.
77.   Realm of Caring. *Pediatric Cannabinoid Dosing Guidelines*. Available from: http://www.theroc.us/images/PediatricGuidelines.pdf.

Chapter 5 – Finding a quality CBD source

For most of us savvy shoppers, we look at any product that we are going to purchase or buy in terms of its quality. There are of course times that we might put a lower cost ahead of quality, such as when shopping the clearance rack or when purchasing soft drinks for the company party. For the most part, however, few of us will sacrifice safety in place of quality. We might not necessarily invest in only 'organic' produce or 'free range' chicken due to the additional costs associated with those products, but at the same time few of us will likely order chicken at a restaurant with an unfortunate reputation for serving undercooked meats.

In the vast majority of patients, CBD is taken as a health product. As such, it is designed to either improve some aspect of our health or perhaps help in the prevention of an unfortunate condition. Given that we are both putting CBD in our body and utilizing it for health benefits, it behooves us as patients to ensure that what we are taking is of a reputable quality. As discussed in an earlier chapter, we can't physically 'see' the CBD in the lines of bottles for sale on the shelf. Consequently, we are left to trust that the CBD was manufactured using quality techniques designed to limit potential contaminants and ensure that the labeled amount is actually present within the sample. Only then can we be assured that we are giving ourselves the best opportunity to reap the benefits of CBD. When it comes to your health, even the 'little things' can make a significant difference, and your CBD is no different. Therefore, this chapter focuses on outlining some of the factors for you to evaluate when choosing a particular CBD product, with the intent of arming you with important information that can help you choose the best CBD for your health.

What to look for in your CBD

Because you are likely choosing to use CBD as a means to improve your health, it's no time to sacrifice on quality. Therefore, seek out the highest quality of CBD that you can find for your chosen route of administration (e.g. oral, topical, etc.). The surge of CBD interest in recent years – combined with the relatively simple extraction procedures that can be used to produce CBD – has allowed for a wealth of 'suppliers' to flood the market with product. While many of these suppliers are reputable, others are no doubt after the easy money that can often be found among patients seeking to use CBD as a potential 'last resort' treatment. Low-cost CBD is most likely the quickest to get on the market, particularly if it went through the extraction process and then went immediately into a bottle without much quality control analysis. With little extra expense involved for the producer, minimally processed CBD can be sold at a low cost. Unfortunately, without subsequent analysis of the product (which would incur additional cost) to include actual CBD content as well as possible contaminants, a patient is left to the mercy of the extraction process's efficiency along with the assumption that what is being sold does indeed contain a viable amount of CBD.

So how can you go about determining what is 'high quality' CBD from all the available options? After all, no manufacturer is going to openly admit that their product is sub-par or of a less-reputable source. As a consumer, being able to weed through the vast amount of advertising ploys can be challenging, but once you know what to look for, it can make you a much more educated consumer. For starters, don't rely much on patient testimonials. Often, CBD sites will post a few '5 star' reviews with commentary that extols the benefits of the product. In reality, no manufacturer who posts a select few reviews is going to list any of the poor reviews; instead, they'll weed through the reviews to find a few tidbits of positive commentary to post. After all, how do you know that those five positive reviews they posted on their site weren't countered by 720 negative reviews? And, were individuals paid or 'remunerated' for posting a positive review? If so, the person posting the review certainly had reason to post an overly positive review that may not have included any particularly negative aspects for fear of it costing them their financial reward.

Next, look for 'third-party' or 'independent lab' analysis of the extract. If a site says that they analyze every batch of their own extract, that might indeed be true, but there may be some bias involved with what they reveal, especially in holding back any specific information such as contaminants found in the sample. Remember, a label stating 'independently analyzed' is not the same as having a manufacturer actually reveal the analysis' results, so look for both the analysis used (i.e. independent, third-party, etc.) and the actual analysis results. Similarly, a phrase such as "guaranteed to have 30mg of CBD per dose" is not the same as saying "free of contaminants" or "harvested from plants certified free of pesticides", as being free from contaminants does not also indicate the actual quantity of CBD in the product. Always, always, seek out manufacturers

117

who can provide certified analyses for each production run of CBD that they produce.

While not specific to quality of the product, it can be important as a consumer to evaluate the credentials and experience of the manufacturer or seller. Is he or she trained with years of experience working with cannabinoids or are they someone looking for a side hustle who only learned of CBD three weeks prior, after a friend's recommendation? Can they answer questions specific to manufacturing processes or harvesting procedures, or can they only tell you that every possible medical condition you have is certain to respond positively to CBD? Do they understand the physiology of the endocannabinoid system? Do they understand their state's CBD regulations? If you have questions in these areas, as a customer you should expect open and honest answers – not to mention *correct* answers. Therefore, look for credibility in your CBD supplier or seller, particularly someone who is trained in *all* aspects of CBD who can in turn provide knowledgeable answers to your questions. After all, along with your medical provider, your CBD supplier is aiding you in making decisions about your health. Therefore, there should be an expectation on your part that he or she is basing their decisions on knowledge of the product rather than simply rehashing a canned response.

Another important area to discuss with your CBD supplier as well as your healthcare provider is specific to the most beneficial route of administration for your CBD. We discussed this topic earlier, but it's worth rehashing in a discussion about making informed choices about your CBD. Certain routes of administration such as inhalants or sublingual (under the tongue) application will result in rapid CBD entry into the bloodstream. For certain medical conditions, topical application may be preferred. Edibles or pill/tablet routes of administration will result in delayed entry into the bloodstream due to their having to be processed by the digestive system yet may allow for a higher dose. When it comes to the recommended route of administration, factors such as how long it can take for the CBD to reach your tissue of interest (e.g. inner ear), your costs for the different CBD preparations, and your medical provider's recommendations should all play into the final decision.

It is also worthwhile to evaluate the different extraction methods to determine which method you are comfortable with. For example, ethanol-based extraction has the potential to denature the CBD molecule due to the heat required. Consequently, some have argued that ethanol extraction is not a preferred method[1] compared to CBD extracted via CO_2, as CO_2 extraction largely avoids heat and reduces the possibility of lessening the CBD quality. Some forms of CO_2 extraction do still use solvents though, which could affect a patient's decision to use CBD that undergoes such CO_2 extraction procedures[2]. Temperature matters during the extraction process, yet individual manufacturers may employ different extraction temperatures. Therefore, a question along the lines of *Does the manufacturer use ethanol extraction, and if so, at what temperature* would be a valid question to ask your CBD supplier.

Because quality is important in health-related products, it has been recommended for patients to seek out CBD that was extracted from products certified as organic by the U.S. Department of Agriculture[1]. Doing so can not only help ensure a higher quality plant but also helps reduce the risk of contaminants such as herbicides or pesticides which have been found in CBD products[3]. Using organic-based CBD is of particular importance given that cannabis is known to be prone to absorbing heavy metals, pesticides, and other soil contaminants[2]. This ability for contaminants to infiltrate the plant has led to recommendations that cannabis crops be tested for contaminants and THC content throughout the growth cycle – not just at harvest[2].

119

Our final point of discussion when looking for high-quality CBD is to seek out CBD that includes a quick response (i.e. "QR") code on the label (Figure 5.1). The QR code can be easily scanned with an app that leads the buyer to a website outlining specific information about the manufacturer, the particular product line of CBD, or even details about the specific CBD you are buying.

Figure 5.1. An example of a QR code that can be found on the label of many CBD products. Using an 'app' on their phone, consumers can scan the QR code to find out important information about the product such as manufacture date, CBD quantity, and source

For example, information that could be presented by a manufacturer includes the source of the cannabis plant (including harvesting practices), the CBD content of the batch used in the product you are buying, testing/analysis procedures, and even the packaging date. While it's largely left up to the manufacturer of a specific CBD product as to what they will include in their QR link, it should be understood that reputable manufacturers would *want* to include an array of information so as to ensure transparency with their customers. Any manufacturer that does not provide such information, or who cannot answer questions specific to areas such as the type of plant source (e.g. marijuana vs. hemp), actual CBD quantity, or analysis techniques, should be considered as questionable by the patient.

A key part of what should be available when scanning the QR code – or perhaps even available at the location from which you purchase CBD – is the manufacturer's 'Certificate of Analysis' that outlines in detail the results of the chemical analysis for a particular CBD batch. In some cases, such as CBD derived from hemp, analysis is not required prior to sale[4]. However, many reputable companies will often seek out testing on their own from third-party laboratories. The state of Indiana could be considered a pioneer in terms of requiring manufacturer transparency as it *requires* all hemp-derived CBD products to include a QR code on their label, with that code in turn leading to information that includes its expiration date, ingredients, and an independent laboratory analysis[5]. Remember, though, that performing this additional testing will incur added costs to the manufacturer, and in most cases these costs will likely be reflected in the final product. You will ultimately have to make your own determination of whether the quality of the CBD justifies any increased cost.

Conclusion

While previous chapters in this book were focused on providing information specific to CBD itself, this chapter focused on what you as a patient should look for in a quality CBD product so as to help yourself to make smart decisions about your CBD. Perhaps the most important thing you can do as a patient is to educate yourself about all aspects of CBD – understanding the characteristics of the plant, identifying the different ways that CBD can be extracted, and knowing the variations that can occur in both CBD itself as well as in the various routes of administration. Furthermore, you will certainly help ensure that you have a quality product by evaluating the Certificate of Analysis to look for not only the true CBD content but also included contaminants such as pesticides or THC. Manufacturers who can both provide you solid answers to your questions and who provide products that can hold up to a thorough analysis should be given priority for receiving your business. And using those products that come from high-quality manufacturers can help ensure that you have a beneficial CBD experience.

Chapter References

1. VanDolah, H.J., B.A. Bauer, and K.F. Mauck. *Clinicians' guide to cannabidiol and hemp oils*. in *Mayo Clinic Proceedings*. 2019. Elsevier.
2. Gill, L., *How to shop for CBD*, in *Consumer Reports*. 2018.
3. Migoya, D., *State recalls 50 Tree of Wellness medical pot products because of pesticide*, in *Denver Post*. 2017.
4. Herrington, A. *The trouble with lab testing in the hemp CBD oil industry*. 2019.
5. State of Indiana, *Senate Enrolled Act No.52*. 2018.

Chapter 6 – The Scientific Process

In the world of healthcare it can be difficult to separate out the facts from the non-facts. Scientific experiments are going on around us at all times, and findings from those experiments are being reported constantly. From one standpoint this is good as we are continually learning new things that will benefit our health. On the other hand, though, constant new findings often lead to results which counter prior results. It can be dizzying trying to stay current, even for health professionals whose job it is to know the most recent research updates. With new treatments such as CBD, however, there is often not a lot of scientific evidence available to keep up with the surge in popularity. Therefore, patients are often left with anecdotes and trying to sort through the mass of personal recommendations that they come across. Some of what patients hear can hold valuable information; other bits and pieces are often nothing more than rumors or flat-out junk science. Even worse is when certain treatments or therapies are nothing more than an attempt by someone to make a quick buck by taking advantage of ill patients who are desperate for help.

To help protect you from the possibility of being taken advantage of or falling for false hopes, this chapter is focused on helping you understand how to evaluate evidence you hear about a product or condition in order to help you determine whether the information is valid and whether you might want to partake in the recommendation. With CBD, its short history as well as its purported widespread benefits can invite wild tales about its effectiveness, even when there is no evidence to support such information. We'll discuss how to better interpret much of what you hear by introducing you to aspects such as the scientific process, research study participants, and how to identify true results versus what tends to be a mere coincidence. With the advent of the internet and social media, patients can often be bombarded with a wide range of recommendations and treatment options. Becoming more informed in how to recognize the good from the bad and the truth from the falsehoods when it comes to methods to improve your health can benefit you immensely as a patient and maximize your chances for successful treatment.

Why we need the scientific process

Science is all about observations. If a researcher designs an experiment, he or she has already predicted an outcome that is commonly known as the *hypothesis*. By observing what happens during an experiment, his or her hypothesis will be supported or rejected. In some cases, hypotheses are relatively simple, such as *if I flip a coin, it will reveal 'heads' 50% of the time.* In such a simple experiment there is pretty much a one-in-two chance that the coin will show 'heads', as there are only two sides to the coin. Therefore, such a hypothesis is quite easy to prove, for if you drop the coin enough times, it's highly likely that heads or tails will occur approximately 50% of the time.

One thing about good science is that it is never permitted to simply *assume* results. For example, you can't assume that since CBD can help reduce inflammation it will also eliminate a headache. As a researcher you still have to test such a hypothesis in order to see if you were indeed correct. After all, there may be some unknown, small factor that influences your experiment. What if, for example, someone handed you a pair of die and told you to roll them 50 times. You might assume that you will have completely random numbers from 2-12 throughout those 50 rolls. What if, however, you found out that when rolled the die came up as a "three" and "four" 84% of the time? Wouldn't that seem a little odd versus the complete randomness that you predicted? If so, your hypothesis of expecting completely random numbers over and over would be refuted. Even though you assumed that the die were standard, an easy experiment revealed that they were actually rigged. Therefore, in science it is critical that you still test your prediction to ensure that there is not some unknown factor influencing the results.

Making predictions using coins or dice are quite simple examples. Things get much more complicated in terms of experiments and predictions when it comes to fields like medicine or psychology. If a researcher designs a drug with the intent for that drug to cure a specific condition, it is relatively simple in concept to design the drug molecule to fit and bind to a specific receptor in the body that should generate an action that the researcher intends. However, it is much more complicated to get that drug molecule to the area of the body it needs to be, or survive the digestive system, or stay in an active form long enough for it to bind to its receptor. In addition, researchers also have to be able to predict any side-effects or unwanted conditions that may result from that drug; otherwise, even if a drug performs its intended duty, too serious of side effects would ultimately prevent its use. Furthermore, they have to show that whatever positive and negative effects occur do in fact occur consistently across several individuals with that condition. It can be a frustrating and difficult process, but it is essential for establishing the 'truth' and the safety specific to a drug or medical treatment.

Unfortunately, establishing all of these factors takes both time and money. A researcher typically has to obtain a grant in order to pay for the facilities, staff, and equipment to design and test their treatment (i.e. drug, machine, etc.) for a specific condition. On top of that, the researcher has to get approval from a board of experts before they are even allowed to begin their experiment, an often drawn-out process that serves to ensure that what the researcher is proposing is both ethical and necessary. And if the process reveals legitimate results, the researcher then has to be able to show that their results can be replicated (i.e. repeated) across a wide variety of individuals of various backgrounds and health statuses, yet another drawn-out process. Once that occurs and there is a clear and safe benefit in using the drug or product, the researcher will most likely be able to start marketing his or her product. When done properly, this process can take years.

In light of the effort required to develop and test a potential treatment effectively, many individuals and companies have decided that it's much simpler to just forego all of the bureaucratic 'nonsense' and post some treatment online that they believe is effective. You often see this in the many vestibular-related social media groups and message boards. The problem with this approach is that there often lacks real evidence that the treatment actually works. Often, such recommendations are made with the purest of intentions – to provide a treatment option for frustrated patients. In many cases, however, the rationale behind recommending an unproven treatment is financial in nature. And, the person selling the treatment often knows that the product has no proof but could result in a potential for financial gain in store for them if they can just convince enough people to buy the product. Most often, it is up to the consumer or patient to be able to determine whether any claims made by the seller are in fact true or just a sales gimmick.

Testing on subjects

To outline why it is important that treatments work across groups of people rather than just a single person, we need to look at what is commonly referred to as a *subject*, or an individual involved in experimental testing. Subjects could be considered the most important aspect of an experiment, and quality research is based upon very precise selection of subjects.

One of the basics in experimental design is the understanding that humans are very similar but very different from each other. Stand two individuals of the same gender, height, and weight next to each other and you might say that they are very similar. But, if you investigate deeper into what you can't see, you might find that one is allergic to a substance, or has high blood pressure, or maybe has an autoimmune disorder. In other words, looking at their outward appearance tells you nothing about particular details that you can't see, such as an underlying medical condition. So, what may be beneficial or safe for one of them might not be the case for both. Therefore, experiments must be comprised of enough subjects to show that a treatment is effect on a range of patients, with the rare exception of treatments designed for a very specific facet of the population (e.g. patients with seizures who do not respond to seizure medication). If a researcher can show that a treatment works for *many* – even though it may not work for absolutely 'everyone' – it can be cause for getting that treatment approved and on the market.

In medicine, when something applies only to a single entity, such as a person, location, or event, it is referred to as a *case*. For example, a flu outbreak at a school after a student returns from a trip would be specific to that school and is not particularly relevant to *all* schools. Therefore, that particular flu outbreak could be considered a case for that school. Research into that school's flu outbreak would be classified as a *case study* or a *case report*. Similarly, if a patient is allergic to, say bacon, that would make his or her situation a case specific to him or her rather than an expected reaction for everyone, as the vast majority of people are not allergic to bacon. Medical treatments apply similarly – if something works for one single patient, it doesn't necessarily mean that it is an effective treatment. Likewise, if one person cannot use a treatment due to an allergy or some other situation, it does not mean that 'all' individuals should not use the treatment. But, if a treatment works for many people in a variety of situations (i.e. a "pool" of individuals), it is much more likely that the treatment truly works.

When it comes to vestibular treatments and 'cures', you can find a wealth of unique options available online. Celery juice, ear candling, and beet juice are just a few of the many that I have observed in social media groups. CBD is certainly another. Expect, however, that most of these treatments have not only failed to go through the experimental design process as described earlier, but you will also likely find little evidence of consistent effects. Product descriptions may highlight a testimonial or two, but the question you as the patient and consumer have to ask yourself is whether that testimonial is valid and whether that positive comment is worth you purchasing the product. After all, it's no secret that people can get paid to make positive comments about a product.

To outline how a useless product can seem to some consumers to be a miracle cure, we can use the classic example of an old phone scam that perfectly outlines how people can fall for false promises. Say you are a swindler and you are needing some cash. You call 40 people, 20 to whom you tout a new, 'hot' stock "A" and 20 to whom you tout stock "B". Stock "A" ends up doing poorly, so you never call back that group. But stock

"B" does well, so you call back those people and say "see, I *told* you this stock would do well!". Knowing that your potential victims aren't quite sold on your service, you then tell half of those remaining people to buy stock "C", and half to buy stock "D". But only stock "D" ends up doing well. Therefore, you quickly call back the people you told about stock "D", bragging about your skills as a stock genius and asking if they are finally ready to invest. Given what appeared to be your two hot recommendations, many in the group hand over money to you to invest for them. What the people in that group don't know is that 30 of your 40 original phone calls went unreturned due to a lack of product performance. Unfortunately for them, they are quick to hand you their money to invest – after which you skip town, never to be seen again.

As I mentioned, internet-based vestibular treatment options can work similarly. Sure, a person can tout the effects of a treatment for vestibular migraine, but for how many patients did the treatment *not* work well for? If a $10 treatment works on 20 people but does not work on 80, is that a financial risk? Perhaps not, and depending on the potential harm (hopefully there is none) it may be worth trying if nothing else has worked for a patient. But, what if that rarely successful treatment is a series of steps that take a month to complete, costs $400, and has the same 20% success rate? You might be a bit hesitant to partake in such a treatment, and given the associated cost you certainly should be skeptical.

When skepticism arises, your next step should be to simply investigate the claims made. Who made the claim? If the company is touting their own product or performed their own research on their own manufactured product, red flags – a lot of them – should be raised. If the product was tested independently, such as by a third-party researcher who has no ties to the company, it can greatly improve the validity of the product claims. But putting a product through the testing phase

129

costs money, and it is often much easier to just market the product to desperate people and find a way to convince them that it works. Maybe even pay some consumers to write the aforementioned favorable testimonial which will most likely make it onto the product manufacturer's website. As potential customers look through the website, a bunch of positive reviews makes it tempting to purchase the product. But, isn't that really what effective marketing is supposed to do – convince you to buy a product? As the price you are willing to pay increases, you as the consumer and patient have to carefully decide if the product is worth the risk. Having solid information about how the product was tested can play an important role in your decision.

True effects vs coincidence

Along the same lines of establishing whether a product works on a single patient or is effective across a range of patients, it is also important to evaluate the facts about the treatment's reported effects. For example, say a person goes to a rock concert full of loud, booming speakers, and later that night has a good bit of ringing in his ear. A friend gives him an oil to put in his ear, and when he wakes up, the ringing is greatly diminished. The second day after the rock concert, and after a little bit more oil was applied, the ringing disappeared. Does that mean that the oil fixed his acute tinnitus? Or could it be that he simply didn't have the true chronic-type tinnitus that many individuals suffer from, and therefore it went away quickly on its own?

Given the circumstances, it's highly likely that the rock concert caused temporary tinnitus that resolved itself in a few hours. Therefore, the oil had no real effect at all; rather, it was just pure coincidence that the application of the oil coincided with the natural reduction in tinnitus. But what do you think might happen when a few years later that same person runs into a colleague who is complaining of constant ringing in her ear for the past six weeks? There's little doubt that he'll end up touting the effects of the oil that he is certain stopped his own tinnitus. And given the long-term status of her tinnitus, she'll probably want to give it a try.

This scenario outlines the classic situation where a misinterpretation of effects leads to belief in a treatment that doesn't really work. Unfortunately, with chronic conditions like many of the vestibular disorders we are faced with that can create patients who are desperate for relief, there are individuals that capitalize on this desperation in order to hype treatments that have no realistic chance of working. That is the main reason for my adding this 'introduction to research' to the chapter – to make you as a patient and consumer more aware. Now we'll dig a little deeper into what you should be assessing when it comes to vestibular treatments.

Designing experiments

When science looks for a new treatment, it applies the variable of interest (e.g. CBD) to one group called the experimental group and holds back that variable from a second group known as the control group. Then, differences in outcomes are evaluated between the groups, with the experimental group typically expected to have a favorable outcome. For example, if there was a belief that low iron intake caused tinnitus, it could be *tested* by designing an appropriate experiment. The two groups would be equally comprised of individuals of similar gender and age as well as both duration and severity of tinnitus. In other words, you wouldn't want to apply the new treatment to a group of, say, females, and then use all males in the control group. Rather, you want consistency

131

in the makeup of the subjects between the two groups. Therefore, you would establish each group so that they consist of similar individuals (e.g. comparable tinnitus duration, gender, age, etc.). Then, for the experiment you would add the iron supplements to a meal for the experimental group while supplying the same meal to the control group, but without the added iron supplement. As long as everything else stays the same, any consistent results occurring in the experimental group (such as an improvement in the majority of the group's tinnitus symptoms after consuming the additional iron) should be expected to be due to the treatment, and not random coincidence. If there is no improvement in the experimental group after the additional iron intake, it could be reasonably determined that the treatment of iron supplementation has no effect.

We discussed how the makeup of the experiment and control group is important. If, as mentioned, the groups are not made of similar individuals, you would effectively be comparing apples to oranges and therefore, any results you obtain from the experiment would have no real validity. Besides physical makeup such as age and gender, similarity in symptoms between groups is important as well. For example, if you had one group that reported having a low hum for six months and another group had debilitating high-pitched tinnitus for at least ten years, keeping them separated into individual experimental and control groups would result in a major study design flaw. However, if you *mixed* the groups so that some people with short-term and others with long-term symptoms and severity were in the same group, that would be acceptable as it creates a "pool' of subjects of similar conditions between the experimental and control groups.

It is also strongly recommended that the groups are comprised of enough people to capture the possible variations in the condition (i.e. tinnitus) that could affect the results. Do the groups capture all severities of tinnitus, or just a specific one or two types? Is the long-term group all taking a certain medication? Have they had a medical procedure or a condition such as a head injury? If so, these particular situations become *confounders* if they can influence the experiment's results. Say, for example, that ¾ of the people in the aforementioned experimental group were also taking an 'anti-tinnitus supplement' that unbeknownst to anyone actually interfered with iron absorption. If those same people then took the iron supplement, the iron would have no chance to exert its potential effects on tinnitus due to the interference of the anti-tinnitus supplement. Therefore, the experiment's results may end up showing that only some of the people in the experimental group had an improvement in their tinnitus after taking an iron supplement. If those same people were also the ones that were *not* taking the anti-tinnitus supplement, it would make the experiment's results look as though the iron was not very effective when in fact the iron was being prevented from working consistently in the experimental group because some participants were taking the anti-nausea supplement. Such a situation outlines how study design is vital and must include aspects such as ensuring that the group's subjects are properly selected and screened, and confounding factors (such as some subjects taking a certain supplement) are controlled.

This may seem like a lot of detail for a vestibular patient interested in CBD to be worried about, but truth be told, these concepts should be essential before trying out *any* particular treatment. Most pharmaceutical medications have already gone through this process and should leave you little worry as to how they were developed. The bigger issue specific to effectiveness lies with supplements and – perhaps more importantly – online claims. If an individual or company is not willing to discuss how they arrived at their marketing claims such as *"reduced sensation of 'vertigo' severity by 50%"*, it should immediately raise

133

questions for anyone considering the treatment. For example, questions should be raised such as "Reduced in what population?" "How long was the treatment given?" "Did they have any other treatments or do anything else simultaneously?" "How and when was the vertigo measured?" The more questions that can be answered legitimately, the more credibility the product gains. Do not be afraid to challenge any claim or product before you spend money on it!

There are certainly times when a treatment may only be tested and shown successful on a particular type vestibular patient such as females, or only when patients have had sensations of dizziness for less than a month, and that limited evidence is perfectly acceptable if the product is marketed as such. In those cases, it is fine to report the findings as long as the success is also reported to be *limited* to that particular population. Remember – assuming is not permitted when it comes to 'assuming' that a treatment reported in one group will apply similarly to another. In other words, if a treatment has not been tested on a particular type of vestibular patient (within reason, of course), it cannot be assumed that the treatment will work until that factor is addressed using a reputable scientific study. So, if a treatment is shown to reduce the incidence of vertigo attacks in postmenopausal vestibular migraine female patients, it cannot be assumed that the product will also work equally well in males until that has been shown with a proper experiment.

What is all of this saying? Simple – it is recommended that you first look for treatments that have gone through the rigor of scientific testing if you're going to spend money on the treatment. CBD brings in a unique aspect given that it is quite new yet also has the issue of federal regulations preventing much interest in it being studied. Still, CBD will not likely be your *first* treatment option for an ongoing vestibular disorder given that vestibular therapy, diet, and stress-relief techniques have been shown to be quite beneficial at lessening the effects of many vestibular conditions. There is actually much, much more that we could discuss regarding the scientific process and how it applies to vestibular treatments, as we have just skimmed the surface. But, what we have discussed should help you to ask questions and read with more detail the evidence behind treatments that you encounter.

If there is no clear evidence or indication of a treatment's proof outside of personal claims, you can still certainly try the product, but know that there are risks to your health as well as your wallet that should be addressed first. At the same time, I am cognizant that there is no cure yet for many vestibular conditions and as such, the cure remains 'out there' somewhere. As we continue to eliminate ineffective treatments, we strengthen the pool of effective options while also expanding our search into promising new areas. When considering an alternative treatment for your own condition – even if that treatment involves CBD – consider the financial cost, any physical risk including side effects, and the evidence that exists for the treatment. The degree of proof that is required in order to use a particular treatment is ultimately left up to you.

Summarizing the scientific process

In drafting out this book I wanted to be sure to include this chapter because it is important to me as an author that you are aware of how to wade through the vast amount of information that you will be presented with specific to vestibular treatments. As a former researcher, I am immediately skeptical of any claim presented as anecdotal rather than based in the scientific process; that is just the effect of my years of research-based training and it is not exactly right or wrong as a belief. To a vestibular sufferer, though, living with the invasiveness of the constant perception of motion may lead them to try *anything* regardless of the purported benefits. And in many cases this can be ok as long as it doesn't cause physical or financial harm to you. But it can also lead to wasted time and false hope if you're not careful, and false hope often leads to repeated bouts of disappointment and/or depression as yet another hopeful cure falls flat. So, take the information you learned in this chapter and always be sure to perform your own level of evaluation of a treatment's effectiveness. If you happen to find something that works for you, by all means use it! It certainly doesn't *have* to have gone through the research process, particularly if it's a natural product (e.g. spice, herb, CBD). But if you are actively looking for treatments and read a claim online, look for the sources or research used to establish that claim. If you are told of a treatment that can help, ask what it is about the product that works along with how it works better than other available options. Being diligent about these claims can help ensure that you are making valuable progress toward a beneficial treatment that can help reduce your own symptoms.

Conclusion

There has been very little research conducted in the area of vestibular-based disorders and their response to CBD. At the same time, CBD is a relatively new treatment option in medicine, and given the rush of attention it has received in the past couple of years it's quite possible that the research process just hasn't had time to go through the lengthy procedures necessary to produce quality studies. Unfortunately, the hype surrounding CBD has grown immensely, often with little evidence for the many claims that appear online specific to how to treat or even cure many of the vestibular disorders. As a vestibular patient, use the information in this chapter to help you weed through the many treatment recommendations you will come across, many of which have been proven over time yet many more that are really nothing more than personal opinion – the result of one patient's success. Remember, though, that the potential for harm along with the financial investment should be key factors in your decision. If there is little personal risk, it may be worth trying; however, much like treatment success, risk is often established through experimental research to determine which factors increase one's risk. CBD is certainly not immune to critical review. And although we stated it earlier in the book, it is worth saying again - as a patient you should ask many questions of both your CBD supplier and your medical professional specific to evidence, cost, risk, route of administration, and other aspects prior to electing CBD as a treatment option. Being informed can be the best option you give yourself as a patient!

Chapter 7 – CBD and Vestibular Conditions

The scientific road to discovery can often be a long and quite drawn-out process. The steps involved in getting approvals, funding, finding appropriate subjects, and then actually conducting the research can take years in order to find a single answer for a specific illness. As a patient afflicted with a debilitating vestibular ailment, it's not unwarranted to expect a fix for your condition *now*. Unfortunately, many vestibular disorders are still poorly understood which in turn means that effective treatments to improve them cannot progress given that a specific target tissue has not been identified. Cannabidiol does offer some promise for many medical conditions, but its impact on vestibular-related ailments remains quite hazy.

In this chapter we'll look at just what the research has revealed specific to CBD's potential influence on some of the more common vestibular conditions. Establishing CBD's true influence can be quite challenging given that it can be difficult to differentiate the many associated complications of vestibular disorders (e.g. anxiety, altered sleep patterns, etc.) from symptoms related to the vestibular condition itself, such as dizziness, nausea, vertigo, etc. Be aware, though, that the findings discussed in this chapter will be limited to known effects of treating some of the more common vestibular conditions with CBD. There is a wealth of information specific to medical marijuana treatment of vestibular-related disorders, but that is outside the scope of this book. Still, even many of the purported effects of medical marijuana treat the ancillary symptoms of vestibular conditions such as anxiety or nausea; however, a reduction in these related effects is not necessarily equivalent to improvement of the particular vestibular condition itself. So while there does appear promise for medical marijuana at treating some vestibular conditions, our focus for this chapter will remain on outlining the research-related effects of CBD. And though there is much anecdotal evidence reported online surrounding CBD's potential influence in this area, we will focus our efforts here on what has been revealed through scientific research studies rather than individual claims.

Tinnitus

Tinnitus is included in this chapter given its widespread prevalence as well as its association with the inner ear. However, it is important to understand that tinnitus is not an actual condition; rather, it is a symptom in the same way that 'pain' is not a medical condition but rather a symptom. Therefore, tinnitus is thought to exist as a result of some other abnormality rather than occurring simply on its own. As such, improvement of tinnitus is likely dependent upon determination of what is causing the tinnitus rather than treating the tinnitus directly.

Tinnitus is a word derived from the Latin *tinnire* ("to ring") and is defined as the perception of sound without a true external source[1]. In other words, a tinnitus patient feels as though they are hearing something even though nothing in the environment around them is generating that perceived 'sound'.

Therefore, the sound patients feel that they are hearing is actually generated internally from some as-yet-undetermined source. This perceived sound can take on many different forms, including ringing, hissing, humming, or buzzing, and can be both intermittent in nature as well as coming in repetitive bursts[2].

Tinnitus can be triggered by several factors. Prolonged exposure to noise is the most common cause, triggering up to 22% of cases[3]. Additional originating events for tinnitus can include head and/or neck injury (17%) and infection (10%), along with other medical conditions (13%) such as disorders affecting the central nervous system[3] (e.g. meningitis) or issues involving cerebral blood flow[4] (e.g. stroke). One's work environment can increase the risk for tinnitus as well. For example, among military veterans, tinnitus has been reported to be the most common service-related condition requiring disability compensation[5]. Psychological factors can also play a role, as tinnitus has been shown to occur in response to stress or other emotional factors[6].

Although tinnitus can occur on its own, it has also been reported in conjunction with other medical conditions of the ear. Ménière's disease, acoustical neuroma, and depression/anxiety[7] have all been reported to involve tinnitus in many cases. Similarly, orthopedic factors such as disorders of the temporomandibular (i.e. jaw) joint can trigger tinnitus[8]. We will discuss many of these associated conditions in a later chapter.

While the onset of tinnitus can have a variety of factors, the actual structural cause of tinnitus is not as well understood. In the majority of cases, tinnitus seems to arise from issues within the cochlea[2, 4]. Particular issues can include lesions brought about by traumatic noise, age-related hearing loss, or pharmaceutical drugs that can be damaging to the structures of the ear[2]. Furthermore, physical changes within the ear, such as growth of a benign tumor on the auditory nerve can also trigger

141

tinnitus[9]. For other patients, however, tinnitus can begin without any specific event that the patient can identify[4]. In these patients it has been theorized that over time an alteration to the components of the auditory system occurred which then generated the effects of tinnitus[2].

CBD and Tinnitus

As far back as 1698, Lemery wrote "Hemp contains much oil, little salt, it is specific for burns, for roaring in the ears, to kill worms"[10]. Interestingly, CB1 receptors are found on cochlear nucleus cells, and no evidence exists for recreational THC use increasing tinnitus after use[11]. CBD can bind to certain receptors known as transient receptor potential vanilloid (TRPV)-4 that are found on inner-ear hair cells[10, 12], and CB1 receptors are located within the cochlear nucleus of the brain[13] which receives neural signals from the inner ear. So in theory, the potential certainly exists for CBD to exert some sort of interaction with the inner ear.

One study did look at how tinnitus may be impacted by the presence of CBD. In rats with sound-induced hearing damage, the presence of tinnitus appeared to increase after receiving a 1:1 ratio of CBD:THC[14]. Of particular interest in this study was that the evidence of tinnitus in those rats appeared to increase *during* the CBD:THC treatment, suggesting that this particular ratio of drug may be responsible for the short-term increase in tinnitus among rats who had been subjected to noise-induced ear trauma. Another study reported that synthetic CB1 receptor agonists, which mimic the effect of cannabinoids, exacerbated tinnitus-related behavior in rats at certain doses[15]. Collectively, these two studies suggest that cannabinoids may serve to worsen, rather than improve, tinnitus. However, it is worth noting that neither animal study looked specifically at CBD alone, nor were the effects of CBD on tinnitus evaluated in humans.

Ménière's disease

Ménière's disease is an illness thought to result from problems with the fluid regulation system of the inner ear. Ménière's patients typically experience an ongoing degree of unsteadiness and ear pressure or fullness intermixed with bouts of acute vertigo, nausea, and vomiting that can last several hours or more. Due in large part to the complexity and sensitivity of the vestibular system, Ménière's remains a complicated disease. While the acute vertigo attacks of Ménière's can be extremely debilitating, those attacks can be followed by months or years of almost no symptoms.

Several theorized causes of Ménière's have been proposed, including body water regulation issues, endolymph reabsorption anomalies, vascular abnormalities, and autoimmune factors. Of these possible causes, fluid regulation in the middle ear is considered to be one of the main triggers of Ménière's[16]. For example, water channels, which regulate the transport of water across membranes, have been implicated as a possible main cause of Ménière's[17]. This theory results from the idea that unexpected reductions or increases in the number of water channels can influence the balance of fluid on each side of a membrane, and any alteration in fluid balance can have negative consequences in the equilibrium system of the ear.

Similarly, some researchers suggest that Ménière's patients have a diminished capacity to regulate fluid within their inner ear[18]. Consequently, fluctuations in the inner ear fluid are not well tolerated in Ménière's patients. This is thought to lead to fluid imbalances that contribute to many of the symptoms encountered by Ménière's patients. Electrolytes such as sodium that are known to play a role in the body's fluid regulation are commonly restricted in Ménière's patients in order to reduce potential fluctuations within the middle ear.

Other theorized causes of Ménière's disease include autoimmune disorders[19], the herpes virus[20], cervical (i.e. neck) disorders[21] and stress[22]. Whereas no definitive cause of Ménière's has been discovered, it is vital that research continues to investigate these and all logical possibilities to determine the potential link and/or similarities between Ménière's and balance-related disorders such as *Mal de Debarquement Syndrome*. At present there remains no cure for Ménière's, though symptoms can often be controlled through the aforementioned sodium restriction, medication, intratympanic steroid injection, and if necessary, surgical procedures on the middle ear.

CBD and Ménière's

At present, no Ménière's-based research has suggested either a beneficial or detrimental response to CBD. The underlying cause of Ménière's has yet to be determined, which in turn makes treatment options difficult as specific therapeutic targets cannot be established. Still, associated effects of Ménière's such as anxiety may show beneficial responses to CBD treatment.

Benign paroxysmal positional vertigo

As we have discussed, one of the most common vertigo conditions seen in primary care is benign paroxysmal positional vertigo (BPPV)[23]. Despite the long name, each word plays a role in describing what occurs with the disease. Most patients with this relatively harmless (benign) condition describe sudden (i.e. paroxysmal) and recurring bouts of vertigo that occur with certain positional-dependent head positions.

The mechanism involved in BPPV is thought to be due to the presence of loose crystals (i.e. otoliths) within the semicircular canals of the ear. As otoliths are not normally present within the semicircular canals, certain head movements cause the loose otoliths to contact the delicate hair cells of the semicircular canals, causing them to trigger and falsely indicate body motion when the head is in particular positions. For example, patients with BPPV often report short bouts of vertigo when looking upwards or rolling over in bed[24]. Furthermore, nausea and vomiting can occur with more severe cases such as *intractable BPPV*.

Diagnosis of BPPV typically involves a thorough medical history and evaluation along with manipulating the head in an attempt to reproduce the symptoms. Most commonly, the Dix-Hallpike maneuver is used to attempt to reproduce the symptoms of BPPV. For this procedure, the patient is seated on a table and their head position is manipulated while the patient is put through a series of specific body positions. Because the otoliths will typically induce nystagmus along with vertigo, the patient's eyes are observed for nystagmus along with any patient-reported vertigo. Results of the Dix-Hallpike test are relatively reliable, being able to correctly identify patients with BPPV 83% of the time while correctly excluding patients without BPPV 52% of the time[23].

For those patients testing positive for BPPV, vestibular rehabilitation and/or canalith repositioning (e.g. Epley maneuver) are relatively successful. Vestibular rehabilitation typically consists of a series of head and/or body motions which may involve fixation of the eye on a single point. Pharmaceutical treatments are not recommended for use in the treatment of BPPV as research has shown no benefit[25]. It is also possible that BBPV symptoms return.

CBD and BPPV

Unlike most vestibular disorders affecting balance and equilibrium, the mechanism involved with BPPV appears to be quite well established as involving loose otoliths within the

145

semicircular canals. The modified Epley maneuver has had tremendous success in treating BPPV by repositioning the otoliths to their proper position within the labyrinth. Because BPPV is the result of physical movement of mal-positioned crystals within the ear, CBD would be expected to have little to no effect on the associated dizziness or vertigo. Consequently, no research appears to have investigated the effect of CBD on BPPV. Intractable BPPV, which is a type of BPPV that does not respond favorably to canalith repositioning, also appears to have no definitive research outlining any benefit or detriment in response to CBD.

Vestibular migraine

Vestibular migraines are among the more common vestibular disorders, affecting up to 1% of the population[26, 27] and up to 11% of patients seeking treatment in dizziness-related clinics[28]. Vestibular migraines are also relatively common in children, having been reported to occur in nearly 3% of children aged 6-12 years of age[29]. Like Ménière's disease, vestibular migraine has no universally accepted definition, which can in turn limit recognition of vestibular migraines in affected patients. Only recently were the diagnostic criteria established which include the following[28].

1. Vestibular migraine
   <u>A</u>. At least 5 episodes with vestibular symptoms of moderate or severe intensity, lasting 5 minutes to 72 hours
   <u>B</u>. Current or previous history of migraine with or without aura according to the International Classification of Headache Disorders (ICHD)
   <u>C</u>. One or more migraine features with at least 50% of the vestibular episodes:

– headache with at least two of the following characteristics: one sided location, pulsating quality, moderate or severe pain intensity, aggravation by routine physical activity

– photophobia and phonophobia

– visual aura

D. Not better accounted for by another vestibular or ICHD diagnosis

2. Probable vestibular migraine

A. At least 5 episodes with vestibular symptoms of moderate or severe intensity, lasting 5 min to 72 hours

B. Only one of the criteria B and C for vestibular migraine is fulfilled (migraine history or migraine features during the episode)

C. Not better accounted for by another vestibular or ICHD diagnosis

The predominant symptoms of vestibular migraine include vertigo in combination with headache, and these two symptoms often occur relatively close to each other[24]. Other symptoms can include transient hearing fluctuations[30], nausea, vomiting, and a sensitivity to motion sickness[28]. Some patients have reported triggering of their migraine in response to dehydration, lack of sleep, or certain foods, but the relationship between these characteristics and vestibular migraines has not been well-studied[28]. Evidence of effective treatment of vestibular migraines is limited. Patients who respond favorably to anti-migraine medication have occurred, but the evidence is lacking as to overall effectiveness[31].

CBD and Vestibular Migraine

Vestibular migraine is one of the newest-recognized vestibular conditions. Whereas the diagnostic criteria for vestibular migraine have been around less than a decade, associated research into CBD's effects on vestibular migraine has not yet been conducted[32]. Furthermore, no studies have been performed on CBD's effect on migraine, though a few studies have evaluated the effect of marijuana and headaches[33].

Persistent Postural-Perceptual Dizziness (PPPD)

As one of the most recently recognized vestibular disorders, our understanding of PPPD is quite limited. At present, no studies have determined the incidence or prevalence of PPPD, though the average patient is reported to be in their mid-40s, with a slightly higher occurrence rate in women[34]. Symptoms of PPPD are subjective in nature and do not exhibit any outward signs, but often include dizziness and/or unsteadiness that can fluctuate in severity[34]. These symptoms are often worsened when the patient has an upright posture[35] and are typically reduced when the patient lies down[34]. Movement, whether active or passive in nature, typically worsens the patient's symptoms, and the speed of the motion tends to correlate to the degree of symptoms that the patient experiences[34]. Patients also note that visual stimuli, such as shadows aligning a roadway or walking down a grocery store aisle can often exacerbate symptoms.

The cause of PPPD remains unknown, but given the relative 'newness' of PPPD as a medical condition, there will likely be an increase in the amount of research directed toward it. Most patients exhibit the symptoms of PPPD after a particular vestibular event such as BPPV or vestibular neuritis[36], though a vestibular event is not required, as stress, anxiety[36], or even head trauma can trigger the effects of PPPD[37]. This prior vestibular event may cause some degree of difficulty in allowing the brain to separate out the multiple balance and proprioception inputs which in turn leads to chronic dizziness[38].

Though no cure for PPPD exists at present, several treatment options have been shown effective for reducing symptoms. Vestibular rehabilitation[39], cognitive behavioral therapy[40], medication[41], and nerve stimulation have all shown promise at treating the symptoms of PPPD[42].

CBD and PPPD

At present there is no research that outlines any effectiveness for CBD in treating PPPD. That being said, PPPD does have a significant anxiety component which may show some improvement in response to a proper CBD dose. Any reduction in anxiety may aid in lessening the overall symptoms of PPPD.

Vestibular neuritis

Vestibular neuritis is associated with vertigo, nausea, vomiting, and imbalance, and is thought to be due to viral inflammation of the vestibular nerve[43]. The condition is considered to be acute as symptoms typically last from a few days to several weeks, but up to half of patients suffering from vestibular neuritis can experience symptoms for a much longer time[44]. Vestibular neuritis has been reported to account for nearly 10% of all dizziness-related medical visits[45]. Interestingly, viral epidemics trigger an increased incidence of vestibular neuritis, lending evidence to its likely inflammatory origins[46].

Patients exhibiting vestibular neuritis will present with acute, severe vertigo[24]. The most severe attacks can last for one to two days and then gradually subside over the following weeks. Motion may worsen the vertigo, and some patients experience nausea and vomiting in conjunction with the vertigo[24]. Additional symptoms often include nystagmus along with a walking pattern in which the patient tends to lean toward the affected ear's side.

Treatment of vestibular neuritis includes symptomatic care along with vestibular rehabilitation, which can begin as soon as tolerable after cessation of immediate symptoms[24]. Vestibular rehabilitation has been reported to be successful when compared against no therapy[47]. If vestibular neuritis is severe, short-term hospitalization may be required until the patient is able to recover[24].

CBD and vestibular neuritis

There is not at present any research directed at investigating whether CBD is an effective treatment for improving vestibular neuritis.

Acoustic Neuroma

Acoustic neuromas, or 'vestibular schwannomas', are slow growing benign tumors[48] of the eighth (vestibulocochlear) nerve[49]. The tumor is slow-growing, but can interfere with other structures of the inner ear[50]. With an incidence of 1 in 100,000, acoustic neuromas are quite rare and mainly affect older adults[50]. The most common symptoms of acoustic neuroma include tinnitus as well as hearing loss in the affected ear[50]. Up to 15% of patients do not experience hearing loss or tinnitus but do report vertigo, and that vertigo often results in them tending to drift to one side.

Because they are rather slow-growing, treatment for an acoustic neuroma can range from conservative methods such as simple long-term observation to the more intensive use of radiation[51] and/or surgical removal[49, 52].

Similar to BBPV, the symptoms associated with acoustic neuroma are linked to a physical event which in this case is the presence of a large tumor that compresses a nerve highly involved in balance and equilibrium. Likely due to the clear source of symptoms associated with acoustic neuroma and the effectiveness of the multiple treatment options available, there is currently no associated research into the effectiveness of CBD in treating acoustic neuroma.

Conclusion

Because it has only been gaining attention for the past decade or so, CBD and its associated research is still in its infancy. When coupled with the fact that vestibular conditions such as vestibular migraine and PPPD are also less than a decade old, it can help outline why little is known specific to the effects of CBD on vestibular-related conditions. Further adding to the issue is that the true underlying cause of many vestibular conditions has yet to be established. Therefore, researchers are unable to know which specific tissue type to study in order to establish specific CBD-related targets. At present, only CBD's effect on tinnitus has been studied directly, yet the findings of a potential increase in tinnitus have only been shown in animals and under very specific parameters (e.g. 1:1 CBD:THC ratio). Still, tinnitus is a symptom rather than an actual medical condition. Other true vestibular conditions such as Ménière's disease or PPPD have yet to receive dedicated attention within the research specific to CBD's potential influence. Consequently, without the benefit of sound scientific research we are largely left to put our faith in patient claims and anecdotal evidence for CBD's effectiveness in treating vestibular disorders.

Chapter References

1. Swain, S.K., et al., *Tinnitus and its current treatment—Still an enigma in medicine.* Journal of the Formosan Medical Association, 2016. **115**(3): p. 139-144.
2. Langguth, B., et al., *Tinnitus: causes and clinical management.* The Lancet Neurology, 2013. **12**(9): p. 920-930.
3. Henry, J.A., K.C. Dennis, and M.A. Schechter, *General review of tinnitus: prevalence, mechanisms, effects, and management.* Journal of speech, language, and hearing research, 2005. **48**(5): p. 1204-1235.
4. Møller, A.R., *Tinnitus: presence and future.* Progress in brain research, 2007. **166**: p. 3-16.
5. Yankaskas, K., *Prelude: noise-induced tinnitus and hearing loss in the military.* Hearing research, 2013. **295**: p. 3-8.
6. Hinton, D.E., et al., *Tinnitus among Cambodian refugees: relationship to PTSD severity.* Journal of traumatic stress, 2006. **19**(4): p. 541-546.
7. McKENNA, L., R.S. HALLAM, and R. HINCHCLIFFEf, *The prevalence of psychological disturbance in neuro-otology outpatients.* Clinical Otolaryngology, 1991. **16**(5): p. 452-456.
8. Saldanha, A.D.D., et al., *Are temporomandibular disorders and tinnitus associated?* CRANIO®, 2012. **30**(3): p. 166-171.
9. Lee, S.H., et al., *Otologic manifestations of acoustic neuroma.* Acta oto-laryngologica, 2015. **135**(2): p. 140-146.
10. Pertwee, R.G., *Handbook of cannabis.* 2014: Oxford University Press, USA.
11. Han, B., J.C. Gfroerer, and J.D. Colliver, *Associations between duration of illicit drug use and health conditions: results from the 2005–2007 national surveys on drug use and health.* Annals of epidemiology, 2010. **20**(4): p. 289-297.
12. Lowry, C., S. Lightman, and D. Nutt, *That warm fuzzy feeling: brain serotonergic neurons and the regulation of emotion.* 2009, Sage Publications Sage UK: London, England.
13. Herkenham, M., et al., *Characterization and localization of cannabinoid receptors in rat brain: a quantitative in vitro autoradiographic study.* Journal of Neuroscience, 1991. **11**(2): p. 563-583.
14. Zheng, Y., P. Reid, and P.F. Smith, *Cannabinoid CB1 receptor agonists do not decrease, but may increase acoustic trauma-induced tinnitus in rats.* Frontiers in Neurology, 2015. **6**: p. 60.

15. Zheng, Y., et al., *The effects of the synthetic cannabinoid receptor agonists, WIN55, 212-2 and CP55, 940, on salicylate-induced tinnitus in rats.* Hearing research, 2010. **268**(1-2): p. 145-150.

16. Minor, L.B., D.A. Schessel, and J.P. Carey, *Meniere's disease.* Current opinion in neurology, 2004. **17**(1): p. 9-16.

17. Ishiyama, G., I. Lopez, and A. Ishiyama, *Aquaporins and Meniere's disease.* Current Opinion in Otolaryngology & Head and Neck Surgery, 2006. **14**(5): p. 332-336.

18. Rauch, S.D., *Clinical Hints and Precipitating Factors in Patients Suffering from Meniere's Disease.* Otolaryngologic Clinics of North America, 2010. **43**(5): p. 1011-1017.

19. Kangasniemi, E. and E. Hietikko, *The theory of autoimmunity in Meniere's disease is lacking evidence.* Auris Nasus Larynx, 2018. **45**(3): p. 399-406.

20. Vrabec, J.T., *Herpes simplex virus and Meniere's Disease.* The Laryngoscope, 2003. **113**(9): p. 1431-1438.

21. Bjorne, A., A. Berven, and G. Agerberg, *Cervical Signs and Symptoms in Patients with Meniere's Disease: A Controlled Study.* CRANIO®, 1998. **16**(3): p. 194-202.

22. Söderman, A.C.H., et al., *Stress as a Trigger of Attacks in Menière's Disease. A Case-Crossover Study.* The Laryngoscope, 2004. **114**(10): p. 1843-1848.

23. Hanley, K., *Symptoms of vertigo in general practice: a prospective study of diagnosis.* Br J Gen Pract, 2002. **52**(483): p. 809-812.

24. Wipperman, J., *Dizziness and vertigo.* Primary Care: Clinics in Office Practice, 2014. **41**(1): p. 115-131.

25. Bhattacharyya, N., et al., *Clinical practice guideline: benign paroxysmal positional vertigo.* Otolaryngology--Head and Neck Surgery, 2008. **139**(5_suppl): p. 47-81.

26. Cherchi, M. and T.C. Hain, *Migraine-associated vertigo.* Otolaryngologic Clinics of North America, 2011. **44**(2): p. 367-375.

27. Neuhauser, H., et al., *Migrainous vertigo Prevalence and impact on quality of life.* Neurology, 2006. **67**(6): p. 1028-1033.

28. Lempert, T., et al., *Vestibular migraine: diagnostic criteria.* Journal of Vestibular Research, 2012. **22**(4): p. 167-172.

29. Abu-Arafeh, I. and G. Russell, *Paroxysmal vertigo as a migraine equivalent in children: a population-based study.* Cephalalgia, 1995. **15**(1): p. 22-25.

30. Johnson, G.D., *Medical management of migraine-related dizziness and vertigo.* The Laryngoscope, 1998. **108**(S85): p. 1-28.

31.   Fotuhi, M., et al., *Vestibular migraine: a critical review of treatment trials.* Journal of neurology, 2009. **256**(5): p. 711-716.

32.   American Headache Society. *Migraine and CBD Oil: Doctor Q&A With Stephen Silberstein, MD, FACP, FAHS.*

33.   Baron, E.P., *Comprehensive review of medicinal marijuana, cannabinoids, and therapeutic implications in medicine and headache: what a long strange trip it's been....* Headache: The Journal of Head and Face Pain, 2015. **55**(6): p. 885-916.

34.   Staab, J.P., et al., *Diagnostic criteria for persistent postural-perceptual dizziness (PPPD): consensus document of the committee for the classification of vestibular disorders of the bárány society.* Journal of Vestibular Research, 2017. **27**(4): p. 191-208.

35.   Staab, J.P., *Chronic subjective dizziness.* CONTINUUM: Lifelong Learning in Neurology, 2012. **18**(5): p. 1118-1141.

36.   Trinidade, A. and J.A. Goebel, *Persistent Postural-Perceptual Dizziness—A Systematic Review of the Literature for the Balance Specialist.* Otology & Neurotology, 2018. **39**(10): p. 1291-1303.

37.   Popkirov, S., J.P. Staab, and J. Stone, *Persistent postural-perceptual dizziness (PPPD): a common, characteristic and treatable cause of chronic dizziness.* Practical neurology, 2018. **18**(1): p. 5-13.

38.   Lee, J.O., et al., *Altered brain function in persistent postural perceptual dizziness: A study on resting state functional connectivity.* Human brain mapping, 2018. **39**(8): p. 3340-3353.

39.   Staab, J.P., *Behavioral aspects of vestibular rehabilitation.* NeuroRehabilitation, 2011. **29**(2): p. 179-183.

40.   Edelman, S., A.E. Mahoney, and P.D. Cremer, *Cognitive behavior therapy for chronic subjective dizziness: a randomized, controlled trial.* American journal of otolaryngology, 2012. **33**(4): p. 395-401.

41.   Yu, Y.-C., et al., *Cognitive behavior therapy as augmentation for sertraline in treating patients with persistent postural-perceptual dizziness.* BioMed research international, 2018. **2018**.

42.   Palm, U., et al., *Transcranial direct current stimulation (tDCS) for treatment of phobic postural vertigo: an open label pilot study.* European archives of psychiatry and clinical neuroscience, 2019. **269**(2): p. 269-272.

43.   Schuknecht, H.F. and K. Kitamura, *Vestibular neuritis.* Annals of Otology, Rhinology & Laryngology, 1981. **90**(1_suppl): p. 1-19.

44. Perols, J.B., Olle, *Vestibular neuritis: a follow-up study.* Acta oto-laryngologica, 1999. **119**(8): p. 895-899.

45. Neuhauser, H.K. and T. Lempert. *Vertigo: epidemiologic aspects.* in *Seminars in neurology.* 2009. © Thieme Medical Publishers.

46. Baloh, R.W. and V. Honrubia, *Clinical neurophysiology of the vestibular system.* 2001: Oxford University Press, USA.

47. Hillier, S.L. and M. McDonnell, *Vestibular rehabilitation for unilateral peripheral vestibular dysfunction.* The Cochrane Library, 2011.

48. Nikolopoulos, T.P., et al., *Acoustic Neuroma Growth: A Systematic Review of the Evidence.* Otology & Neurotology, 2010. **31**(3): p. 478-485.

49. McLaughlin, E.J., et al., *Quality of Life in Acoustic Neuroma Patients.* Otology & Neurotology, 2015. **36**(4): p. 653-656.

50. Rosahl, S., et al., *Diagnostics and therapy of vestibular schwannomas–an interdisciplinary challenge.* GMS current topics in otorhinolaryngology, head and neck surgery, 2017. **16**.

51. McClelland, S.I., et al., *Impact of Race and Insurance Status on Surgical Approach for Cervical Spondylotic Myelopathy in the United States: A Population-Based Analysis.* Spine, 2017. **42**(3): p. 186-194.

52. Fusco, M.R., et al., *Current practices in vestibular schwannoma management: A survey of American and Canadian neurosurgeons.* Clinical Neurology and Neurosurgery, 2014. **127**: p. 143-148.

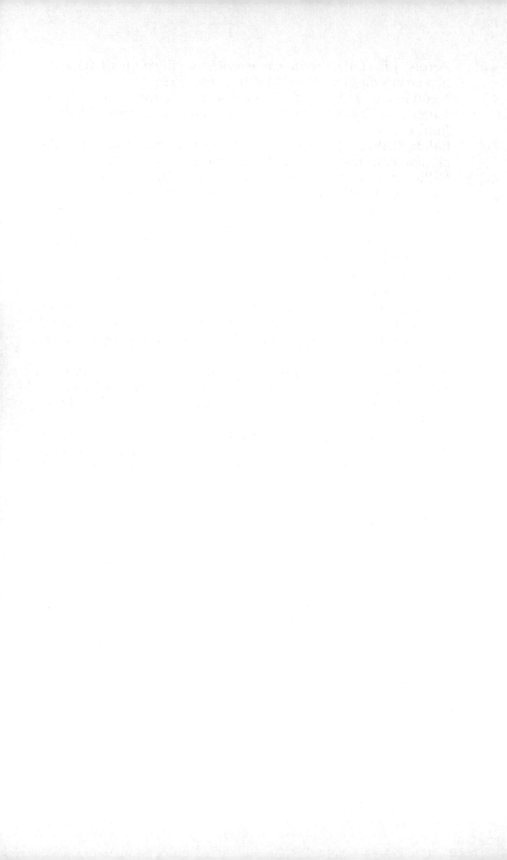

Conclusion

This book was written with the intent of providing you as a vestibular patient an introduction into the world of CBD, with particular emphasis on understanding the mechanisms behind how CBD works as well as how CBD may benefit you as a patient. Certainly, this book could have been produced as a 10-page pamphlet telling you what to look for or how to take CBD, but I think that there are plenty of those already available, and truth be told I personally don't feel that *telling* you specific information holds the same value as providing you a broad aspect of information that you can then use to help you develop and make your own decisions. Given the variability in symptoms that can exist between vestibular patients – even those who have the same condition – a 'one size fits all' approach isn't likely to have much success. Therefore, I feel that educating you as a patient can provide you a much greater opportunity for success than simply telling you which CBD to take for your particular condition.

As a vestibular patient myself, I've been through the range of emotions and symptoms that so many of us have to deal with. The cancelled plans due to an attack, the agonizing silence that can make your tinnitus seem overwhelming, or the hours of nausea and vertigo that can leave you lying in bed waiting for the misery to end. And of course that all-too-familiar mindset that you are powerless to the randomness of attacks. Having lived with some degree of vestibular issues for nearly 20 years, I know too well of all the 'quick fix' recommendations that friends and family offer despite having no true understanding of either the vestibular disorder itself or just how disabling the disorder can be. Even social media, which under the right circumstances can bring us together with others who suffer similarly, can at times lead us down the road of frustration as we are presented with many 'miracle cures' that one or a few people claim led to the end to their vestibular issues.

CBD's relatively short history in the realm of science and medicine has created quite a predicament for patients. On the one hand, most information relating to CBD is only a few years old at most which makes it highly relevant in the medical field. Often, patients are left with information that is decades old, leaving open the question of whether it still applies, or whether more valid information has become available since. On the other hand, though, CBD's short history has prevented it from receiving the research attention afforded to many other treatments including medication. This in turn has contributed to much of the speculation that exists specific to CBD's purported benefits, as many medical professionals want to see hard evidence of benefits rather than relying on speculation or anecdotal reports. Still, CBD has not shown any indication of becoming the latest passing fad as so many other treatment-based products have shown to be. Consistent effects on inflammation, metabolism, and even digestion outline that CBD is influencing certain processes in our body, and our understanding of the endocannabinoid system clarifies just how these processes are being influenced.

In this book we have looked at a variety of topics that you can use to help develop a framework as to how you plan to use CBD to improve your health. In looking at cannabis, we outlined where CBD can be found in the plant as well as how

CBD content can differ across plants. We outlined the endocannabinoid system, looking at how cannabinoids themselves are utilized along with detailing the unique endocannabinoid receptor characteristics. We then discussed several aspects of CBD itself including its design, its safety and side effects, the known effects that CBD has shown in the scientific literature, and how it is extracted from the plant. We then outlined a few aspects to evaluate when making your own CBD decisions. Because of this broad approach, it is my hope that you have the information needed to hold educated and productive talks with your CBD supplier as well as your medical professional.

Hopefully it is just a matter of time before CBD is shown to have consistent therapeutic effects within the vestibular world. Unfortunately, the underlying cause of many vestibular conditions has yet to be revealed. Because we don't know the actual mechanism behind vestibular migraine, PPPD, or other vestibular conditions, it is difficult to develop therapies that can target these debilitating conditions. This lack of understanding of many vestibular disorders is the cause for frustration not only among patients but also for researchers and medical professionals who cannot establish consistent therapies that improve these conditions in patients. CBD may not be a cure-all for each disorder, but there may be promise on the horizon for treating vestibular disorders, particularly those that are suspected to involve inflammation.

Because of the relative 'newness' of CBD and the variation in symptoms and treatment results that can exist across vestibular patients, I included a chapter that helps patients evaluate the evidence when it comes to potential treatments. This chapter was developed from my own experience on social media where I would see almost endless treatment or therapy recommendations for vestibular disorders despite little merit and no scientific basis. But, given that so many patients have already had no improvement with other more established treatments, this lack of a favorable response probably contributed to a desire to try any available option. If those options are legitimate and don't cause harm, I'm all for trying them. But if those treatments require paying money or are hyped from less-than-reputable individuals, it increases the chance that the patient will ultimately experience no real benefits. So, I wrote that chapter to help patients learn how to evaluate the evidence in order to make informed decisions about treatments and products that have a true potential to help them, thereby limiting the chance that they as patients get taken advantage of.

And so, in closing, I hope that you have learned something from this book and that you feel empowered to make decisions about CBD that will improve your health and well-being. Maybe you've decided that CBD is not for you. Or perhaps you feel that CBD is your best option. Regardless of your choice, remember that any treatment is a decision that should involve you and your medical provider – don't stop your current treatment just to try CBD unless that decision is made in conjunction with everyone involved in your healthcare. That may include your physician, family, therapist, and certainly you, among others.

With that being said, I wish you the best on the next phase of your journey with your vestibular condition and, if you choose, with CBD.

Glossary

2-AG – an endocannabinoid that is formed from arachidonic acid and glycerol and binds to the CB1 receptor

Agricultural Hemp – a variety of the Cannabis Sativa L. plant that is comprised of less than 0.3% THC and is grown for industrial purposes

Anandamide – a derivative of arachidonic acid acts as a messenger molecule with involvement in appetite, depression, memory, and fertility

Bioavailability – the amount of the substance that actually enters the bloodstream after the initial dose and is available for use by the body.

Blood Brain Barrier – a barrier that exists between the capillaries and cells of the brain which exists to protect against circulating toxins that could harm the brain, while also allowing vital nutrients to reach the brain

Broad Spectrum – a cannabis product that is includes little to no THC yet contains more than just CBD, such as some minor cannabinoids and terpenes

Cannabidiol (CBD) – the primary non-psychotropic cannabinoid found in hemp

Cannabinoid – one of at least 113 chemical substance produced within the cannabis plant, including cannabidiol

Cannabinoid Receptor Type 1 (CB1) – the receptor for cannabinoids that is predominantly located in the brain and nervous system and to a lesser degree within the lungs, liver, and kidneys.

Cannabinoid Receptor Type 2 (CB2) – the receptor for cannabinoids that is predominantly located within the immune system as well as the spleen and in the gastrointestinal system.

Cannabinoid Receptors – a group of receptors found throughout the body that are responsible for binding to cannabinoids. When cannabinoids bind to their receptors they trigger a series of reactions

Cannabinol (CBN) – a cannabinoid with a very similar chemical composition to THC and thought to primarily bind with the CB2 receptor

Cannabis – a variety of plant also known as hemp, a term reserved for varieties of cannabis cultivated for non-drug use

Cannabis Oil – concentrated extracts that can contain high concentrations of THC

Cannabis Sativa L. – a species of plant that refers to both agricultural hemp and marijuana

CBD Isolate Powder – the purified form of CBD that, after extraction, goes through a purification step to produce a crystalline powder of over 99% CBD

CBD Oil – An extract from the flowering portions of the hemp plant which is combined with other oils and typically contains no THC

CBD Tinctures (Drops) – liquid extracts of hemp that are combined with a carrier (e.g. oil) to be used to deliver CBD as drops or spray

CBD Vape Pods – pre-filled containers that hold CBD and are designed to be used with vape pens

CBD – cannabidiolic-acid, the naturally occurring endocannabinoid produced directly in the cannabis plant

Certificate of Analysis - a document from an analytical testing lab that details out the findings from an analyzed cannabis sample and commonly includes percent composition of cannabinoid, terpenes, and other constituents

CO_2 Extraction – an extraction process that uses supercritical carbon dioxide (i.e. above its critical point) to create effective extracts. CO_2 is the most expensive extraction method, and is widely considered the most effective and safest plant extraction method in the world

Crude Hemp – plant biomass extract that is typically used as the input for a distillation process

Crystallization/Recrystallization – a technique used to purify chemicals

Decarboxylation – removing a carboxyl group from a chemical compound, such as occurs in order to produce the final form of CBD

Delivery Method – the method used to deliver CBD into your body

Distillate Oil – the oil generated from a distillation process, commonly marketed as CBD oil

Dosing – a quantity of medicine or substance to be taken at one time

Endocannabinoid System – the part of the body composed of chemical receptors, enzymes, and endocannabinoids

Endocannabinoids – chemicals produced by the body that target cannabinoid receptors in the brain

Endogenous: originating from within an organism

Entourage Effect – a belief that some or all of the components of the cannabis plant work as a unit in the body

Fatty Acid – a long hydrocarbon chain consisting of a carboxyl group (COOH) at the end

Flavonoids – compounds in plants which give plants their color and assist in prevention of diseases

Full Spectrum – a cannabis product that contains CBD and other cannabinoids (usually THC) as well as terpenes

Hemp – a variety of Cannabis sativa that contains less than 0.3% THC and grown specifically for industrial use

Hemp Oil – the oil extracted from the hemp plant

Hemp Seed Oil – oil pressed from hemp seed that contains no CBD

Homeostasis – a theoretical state of complete balance in the body

Homogeneity – the degree to which multiple units from a group are similar

Industrial Hemp – a variety of cannabis that contains less than 0.3% THC.

Isolate – pure CBD

Marijuana – cannabis leaves and flowers containing over 0.3% THC and used either recreationally or medicinally

Micro-dosing – a dosing where the dose is broken into smaller sizes and taken several times throughout the day

Oral consumption – a method that entails introducing CBD to the body through the mouth and intestinal tract

Phytocannabinoids – one of 113 naturally occurring cannabinoids that are found in the cannabis plant

Psychoactive – property of a substance or compounds that is capable of affecting a person's mindset, personality, or brain function

Solvent Based Extraction – A process which uses an organic solvents such as butane, ethanol, and carbon dioxide to extract cannabinoids

Sublingual – a method that entails introducing CBD to the body through absorption under the tongue

Terpenes – chemicals found in plants that provide their distinctive flavors and scents

Tetrahydrocannabinol (THC) – one of the primary cannabinoids found in cannabis that is associated with psychoactive effects

Topical – a method that entails introducing CBD to the body application to the skin

Transdermal – similar to topical, a method that entails introducing CBD to the body through the mouth

Vaping – the process of inhaling vapor to introduce CBD to the body

Vitamin E – the chemical alpha-tocopherol which is a fat-soluble vitamin that is important for normal cell growth and function

Winterization – a process used after extraction that further purifies a hemp extract by exposing the extract to sub-zero temperature in order to separate out impurities such as waxes

Appendix A. Drug Schedules

According to the Controlled Substances Act, the following are the five classifications of drugs based on their abuse potential, accepted medical application(s), and safety and potential for addiction.

Schedule 1 (I)
- The drug has a high potential for abuse.
- The drug has no currently accepted medical use in treatment in the United States.
- There is a lack of accepted safety for use of the drug under medical supervision.

Schedule 2 (II)
- The drug has a high potential for abuse.
- The drug has a currently accepted medical use in treatment in the United States or a currently accepted medical use with severe restrictions.
- Abuse of the drug may lead to severe psychological or physical dependence

Schedule 3 (III)
- The drug has a potential for abuse less than the drugs in schedules 1 and 2.
- The drug has a currently accepted medical use in treatment in the United States.
- Abuse of the drug may lead to low or moderate physical dependence or high psychological dependence.

Schedule 4 (IV)

- The drug has a low potential for abuse relative to the drugs in schedule 3.
- The drug has a currently accepted medical use in treatment in the United States.

Schedule 5 (V)

- The drug has a low potential for abuse relative to the drugs in schedule 4.
- The drug has a currently accepted medical use in treatment in the United States.
- Drugs in schedule 5 consist primarily of preparations containing limited quantities of certain narcotics.

Let others know!

If you found this or any of Mark's other books informative, *please take the time and post a review online*! Reviews help get exposure for the books and thereby improve the chances that others will be able to benefit from the material as well!

Check out these other books by Mark Knoblauch

A Patient's Guide to Acoustic Neuroma

Living Low Sodium: A guide for understanding our relationship with sodium and how to be successful in adhering to a low-sodium diet

Mal de Debarquement Syndrome: A Comprehensive Patient Guide

Outlining Tinnitus: A comprehensive guide to help you break free of the ringing in your ears

Overcoming Ménière's: How changing your lifestyle can change your life

PPPD: A patient's guide to understanding persistent postural-perceptual dizziness

Professional Writing in Kinesiology and Sports Medicine

Seven Ways To Make Running Not Suck

The Art of Efficiency: A guide for improving task management in the home to help maximize your leisure time

Understanding BPPV: Outlining the causes and effects of Benign Paroxysmal Positional Vertigo

Vestibular Migraine: A Comprehensive Patient Guide

Photo Credits:

Figure 1.1: Roxana Gonzalez/shutterstock.com
Figure 1.2.: Gleti/shutterstock.com
Figure 2.1: Medial Art Inc/shutterstock.com
Figure 2.2: ilusmedical/shutterstock.com
Figure 2.3: designusa/shutterstock.com
Figure 2.4: maxcreatnz/shutterstock.com
Figure 2.5: designusa/shutterstock.com
Figure 3.1: About time/shutterstock.com
Figure 4.1: William casey/shutterstock.com
Figure 4.2: 420MediaCo/shutterstock.com
Figure 5.1: nicemonkey/shutterstock.com

About the Author

Mark is a small-town Kansas native who now lives in a suburb of Houston with his wife and two young daughters. His background is in the area of sports medicine, obtaining his bachelor's degree from Wichita State and his master's degree from the University of Nevada, Las Vegas. After working clinically as an athletic trainer for eight years, Mark returned to graduate school where he received his doctorate in Kinesiology from the University of Houston, followed by a postdoctoral assistantship in Molecular Physiology and Biophysics at Baylor College of Medicine in Houston, TX. He has been employed as a college professor at the University of Houston since 2013.

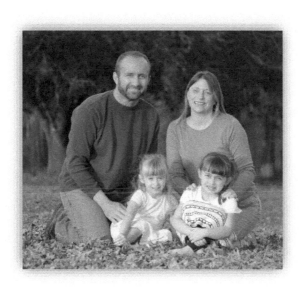

CPSIA information can be obtained
at www.ICGtesting.com
Printed in the USA
LVHW080333120122
708393LV00014B/651